Clinical Skills Review

Clinical Skills Review

Scenarios based on standardized patients

PREPARE FOR
OSCEs
MCCQE II
CFPC certification

EDITED BY

Zu-hua Gao MD, PhD
Christopher Naugler MD, MSc

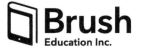

Brush Education Inc.
www.brusheducation.ca
contact@brusheducation.ca

Cover design by Claudia Pompeii, Obsidian Multimedia Corporation (Edmonton, Canada); Cover photo © iStockphoto.com/Marilyn Nieves

Printed and manufactured in Canada

Library and Archives Canada Cataloguing in Publication

Gao, Zu-hua [OSCE & LMCC-II] Clinical skills review : scenarios based on standardized patients / edited by Dr. Zu-hua Gao MD, PhD and Dr. Christopher Naugler MD, MSc. – Third edition.

Includes index. Revision of: OSCE & LMCC-II : review notes / Zu-hua Gao ; Jenika Howell, Karen Naert, Denise Ng, editors. Issued in print and electronic formats. ISBN 978-1-55059-440-9 (pbk.). – ISBN 978-1-55059-453-9 (epub). – ISBN 978-1-55059-483-6 (pdf). – ISBN 978-1-55059-484-3 (mobi)

1. Clinical medicine – Examinations – Study guides.   2. Physicians – Licenses – Canada – Examinations – Study guides.   I. Gao, Zu-hua, editor   II. Naugler, Christopher T. (Christopher Terrance), 1967–, editor   III. Title.   IV. Title: OSCE & LMCC-II

R834.5.G36   2013 616.0076   C2013-903322-X   C2013-903323-8

We acknowledge the support of the Government of Canada
Nous reconnaissons l'appui du gouvernement du Canada | Canada

Contents

List of tables

Introduction

How to use this book

Clinical skills exams—sometimes called "objective structured clinical examinations" or OSCEs—are a rite of passage for all physicians in training. These exams include the MCCQE II and the Certification Examination in Family Medicine in Canada, and equivalent exams in other countries such as the USMLE Step 2 CS in the United States.

This book is designed to help you prepare for these exams. Although simply reading through the cases in this book will be useful, the best way to study for a clinical skills exam is to practice. Groups of 3 or 4 work best, assigned to the following roles:

- **Candidate**: reads aloud a case from the list of cases at the back of the book. Reading aloud ensures that everyone knows the boundaries of the task. The candidate should then "perform the task" by formulating questions to ask the patient, or describing other procedures such as physical examinations or investigations, as required.

- **Examiner**: uses the notes for the case to formulate one or two pertinent questions to ask the candidate and to remind the candidate of any crucial steps they may have missed.

- **Observers**: help debrief the task. We recommend that observers pay particular attention to skills such as: communicating clearly and respectfully; setting appropriate priorities; engaging issues of medical ethics as needed; and resolving clinical situations that require the expertise of specialists.

Work through all the cases in the book in this way, changing roles each time.

Each case has time limit—either 5 minutes or 10 minutes—in keeping with the protocols for the Canadian clinical skills exams. In some instances, in an effort to be comprehensive, the cases set up more tasks than a candidate could realistically accomplish within the assigned time. It is still useful, however, to set a timer or stopwatch for the assigned time, to get a feel for "how long you have."

Take the time to work through all the cases thoroughly and thoughtfully, so start at least a few months in advance of the exam. This will allow you to use each case to its fullest—exploring different issues and questions that each could contain—and allow you to gain some level of comfort and confidence in the face of an otherwise stressful exam.

We have tried to avoid the use of jargon as much as possible. However, in the interests of space we have used a number of abbreviations, and we have listed these in the abbreviations section at the back of the book.

Medicine is famous for the number of mnemonics that students have developed over the years to remember certain aspects of history or management, and we have given these as appropriate throughout the book. Memorizing the most important of these should prove useful in situations where you need to think on your feet.

No book of this nature can ever be "complete." We encourage you to draw from other sources in preparing for your clinical skills exam. In particular, you should be familiar with advanced lifesaving (ALS) protocols, and should review general textbooks in each of the areas in which you will be tested.

Approach to clinical stations at the exam

At the exam, you will encounter clinical stations. Each will have a simulated patient and an examiner. Some stations—those about trauma or cardiac emergencies, for example—may also have a "helper" present such as a nurse.

In general you should ignore the examiner unless they specifically address you.

You should be dressed professionally and you should act professionally. Introduce yourself to the simulated patient and shake their hand if appropriate. If you are asked to perform a physical examination, ask the simulated patient for permission before you start.

Remember that, in a clinical examination like you are facing, the cases you are given to work through will be diagnosable. The examiners will not be trying to trick you. Therefore, if you are handed an ECG to interpret, the diagnosis will likely be straightforward. Furthermore, if you are asked to manage the patient based on the ECG findings, the diagnosis will likely be something that has an advanced life-saving algorithm like an acute myocardial infarction or ventricular fibrillation. Likewise, a lateral C-spine X-ray will be far more likely to show a fracture-dislocation than a rare congenital malformation; a chest X-ray will more likely show a tension pneumothorax than nonspecific findings. You get the picture.

Because the clinical stations aim to test you on relatively common, diagnosable entities, at least some of the examiners' questions are predictable. While this book does not contain all possible scenarios, experience has shown that many stations at the exam will be similar to the scenarios described here.

Unfamiliar scenarios

If you are presented with an unfamiliar scenario, don't panic! Even if you are completely lost, you can still often salvage a station by introducing yourself, acting professionally, performing a history of the presenting complaint, and reviewing symptoms, medications, allergies, family history, and social history. In doing so, you will likely uncover the information that will help you regroup and still do well. If all else fails, ask open-ended questions, such as "Is there anything else you want to tell me?" If you completely flop on a station, regroup and carry on for the next one.

A note on the scenarios

This book unpacks 133 cases organized around the major themes of the Canadian MCCQE II. These themes are logical and the cases are typical— they are on-point preparation for any clinical skills exam. Note that the cases are representative of cases encountered on the Canadian MCCQE II and the Certification Examination in Family Medicine in Canada, but are not direct "remembrances."

General approaches to history taking

History taking is key to many stations in clinical exams, and so to many cases in this book. We present some general strategies for history taking below.

In all cases, it's useful to begin history taking with a quick explanation to the patient, such as "I'm going to ask some questions to get some background information on your health and medical history."

Generally, you should begin with questions about the present illness and then move to past medical history.

HISTORY OF PRESENT ILLNESS

Why are you here today?

When did this symptom/problem start?

FOR PAIN

What is the location?

What kind of pain is it (sharp, dull, throbbing)?

How bad is the pain on a scale of 1 (low) to 10 (high)?

Where does the pain radiate?

When did the pain begin?

What makes the pain worse? What makes it better?

Do you have other symptoms with the pain (e.g., nausea)?

PAST MEDICAL HISTORY

Ask questions to ascertain details about the following areas (mnemonic: **PAM HUGS FOSS**).

Previous presence of the symptom, previous conditions

Allergies

Medicines

Hospitalizations

Urinary changes

Gastrointestinal complains

Sleep pattern

Family history

OB/GYN history

Sexual history

Social history

Note that we describe specific aspects of this sequence in more detail below.

ALLERGY AND MEDICINES HISTORY

What prescription medication do you take? How long and what dosage?

What over-the-counter medications or preparations do you take? How long and what dosage?

Do you have any drug allergies? What was the reaction?

Do you have any nondrug allergies (e.g., food, environmental)? Do you carry an EpiPen?

FAMILY HISTORY

Is there a family history of diabetes?

Is there a family history of high blood pressure?

Is there a family history of heart problems?

Is there a family history of seizures?

Do other diseases run in your family?

OBSTETRICAL/GYNECOLOGICAL HISTORY

It's wise to approach obstetrical and gynecological history taking with particular sensitivity: patients may feel embarrassed.

GYNECOLOGICAL HISTORY

How old were you when you had your first period? (Or—as appropriate—when your breasts began to develop?)

How long is your usual cycle? How many days of bleeding are usual for you? How many pads or tampons do you usually use per day? Are there clots?

Has there been a change in the timing of your cycle?

Do you use birth control pills or hormone replacement therapy?

Have you had a Pap smear before? What were the results of past Pap smears?

What gynecological procedures have you had (e.g., loop electrosurgical excision procedure, hysterectomy)?

Have you had any STDs?

OBSTETRICAL HISTORY

Have you ever been pregnant? If so, how many times?

Have you miscarried? If so, at what stage of pregnancy?

Did you have any problems getting pregnant? Did you use any conception aids?

How many children do you have?

Were there any precipitous deliveries?

Were there any complications in pregnancy (e.g., hypertension, diabetes)?

For each child:

- What was the method of delivery?
- What was the gestational age of the baby?
- What was the baby's birth weight?

SOCIAL HISTORY

What are your living arrangements?

What is your marriage history, family situation?

Do you drink alcohol? How much, how often?

Do you smoke?

Do you use recreational drugs?

PEDIATRIC HISTORY

Keep in mind that, in pediatric cases, patients often don't speak for themselves, or may not speak with clarity.

MATERNAL HEALTH

How is your health today?

How was your health during your pregnancy?

How did the delivery go?

Do you have any concerns about bonding with your baby?

BABY/YOUNG CHILD'S HEALTH

How was your baby's health after the delivery?

What was your baby's birth weight?

What is your method of feeding your baby and how has that been going?

Has your baby had jaundice?

What are your baby's stools like?

How often does your baby have a wet diaper?

ALL CHILDREN'S HEALTH

Do you give your child any supplements (vitamin K, iron) or medications?

Does your child have any allergies that you know of?

Are your child's immunizations up to date?

What is your child's diet like?

What is your child's sleep cycle?

What activities does your child enjoy?

Do you have any concerns about your child in the following areas?

- gross motor or fine motor development
- vision, hearing
- expressive language, comprehension
- social skills, behavior

Medicine

Case 1: Acidemia

A 50-year-old woman presents with acidemia. Please recommend and explain appropriate investigations.

Time: 5 minutes

Investigations

First, specify an ABG test:

- to check pH and confirm acidemia
- to differentiate between respiratory and metabolic acidemia (see Table 1)

Table 1. ABG INTERPRETATION: RESPIRATORY VERSUS METABOLIC ACIDOSIS

TYPE OF ACIDOSIS	ABG INTERPRETATION
Respiratory acidosis	PCO_2 high (opposite to pH)
	HCO_3 high if there is metabolic compensation
Metabolic acidosis	HCO_3 low (in the same direction as pH)
	PCO_2 low if there is respiratory compensation

Next, check if compensation is adequate. Adequately compensated acidosis will produce the following:

- acute respiratory acidosis: PCO_2 increase 10, HCO_3 increase 1 – pH reduce 0.08

- chronic respiratory acidosis: PCO_2 increase 10, HCO_3 increase 3 – pH reduce 0.03
- metabolic acidosis: compensated HCO_3 increase 1, PCO_2 increase 1

Finally, if metabolic acidosis is present, look for a cause by calculating the anion gap: $Na - (Cl + HCO_3)$, which would equal 12 (+/– 2). See Table 2.

Table 2. CAUSES OF METABOLIC ACIDOSIS BY PRESENCE OR ABSENCE OF AN INCREASED ANION GAP

TYPE OF METABOLIC ACIDOSIS	CAUSES
Increased anion gap	(mnemonic: **MUDPILES**)
	Methanol
	Uremia
	Diabetic ketoacidosis
	Paraldehyde/**P**ropylene glycolIsoniazid
	Isopropyl alcohol
	Lactate
	Ethanol/**E**thylene glycerol
	Salicylate
Normal anion gap	Hypoalbuminemia
	Renal tubular acidosis
	Gastrointestinal fistulal
	Ileal loop

Case 2: Elevated liver enzymes

A 55-year-old man comes to your office angry because his insurance turned him down for abnormal liver-function tests. He wants you to "sort out this mistake." His tests to date show very high transaminases, slightly elevated alkaline phosphatase, and normal bilirubin. Please take a history, do a physical exam, provide a differential diagnosis, and recommend investigations.

Time: 10 minutes

History

HISTORY OF PRESENT ILLNESS
When was the blood test done?

Do you have any of the following symptoms?

- fever
- muscle pain
- fatigue
- headache
- cough
- nausea or vomiting
- loss of appetite
- weight loss
- abdominal discomfort
- changes in sense of taste and smell
- itching, jaundice
- bruising

Are these symptoms getting worse or better?

Have you had a blood transfusion recently?

Have you had any recent serious illness or trauma?

Have you been vaccinated against hepatitis?

PAST MEDICAL HISTORY

Have you had any previous treatment for abnormal liver function?

Have you been diagnosed with any of the following?

- cholecystitis
- gallstones
- pancreatitis
- inflammatory bowel disease

What medications do you take (e.g., acetaminophen, isonicotinylhydrazine, methyldopa, steroids, erythromycin, etc.)?

Does your family have a history of any of the following?

- liver failure
- jaundice
- blood disorders
- Wilson disease
- hematochromatosis
- psychiatric disorders
- diabetes
- cystic fibrosis

Do you drink alcohol? How much?

Do you use recreational drugs?

Are you living with a male/female partner? Does your partner have hepatitis or use recreational drugs?

Have you traveled recently? Where?

Have you recently had contact with people with hepatitis?

Physical exam

CATEGORY TO ASSESS	FINDINGS TO NOTE IF PRESENT
Vitals	Fever, hypotension, tachycardia, tachypnea
General condition	Malnutrition, pallor (anemia), jaundice, breath fetor, "bronze diabetes" (hemochromatosis)
Head and neck	Xanthelasmata (chronic cholestasis), parotid swelling (alcohol abuse), bruising, spider nevi, female distribution of body hair, Kayser-Fleisher rings
Neurologic	Ophthalmoplegia, nystagmus, ataxia, lateral rectus palsy, altered mental status, Korsakoff syndrome, retrograde amnesia, impaired learning, confabulation
Hands	Flapping tremor, inability to copy a 5-point star; leukonychia (hypoproteinemia); palmar erythema with wasting; mild finger clubbing, muscle atrophy; Dupuytren contracture
Chest	Gynecomastia, pleural effusion, spider nevi
Abdomen	Dilated veins, collateral; liver and spleen enlargement; ascites; testicular atrophy

Differential diagnosis

See Table 3.

Table 3. DIFFERENTIAL DIAGNOSIS OF LIVER DISEASE

CATEGORY	POSSIBLE ETIOLOGY
Prehepatic (hemolytic)	Red blood cells (RBCs): sickle cell, spherocytes, glucose 6 phosphate deficiency (G6PD), pyruvate kinase deficiency, malaria
	Toxins
	Vascular
Hepatic	Cholestasis: pregnancy, primary biliary cirrhosis, primary sclerosing cholangitis, total parenteral nutrition (TPN)
	Drugs: rifampin, chloramphenicol, contrast
	Congenital decreased conjugation
	Sepsis
Posthepatic	Obstruction: gall stones, stricture (past surgical intervention, atresia), tumor

Investigations

INVESTIGATION CATEGORY	DETAILS
General chemistry	CBC, electrolytes, Cr, urea, glucose
Liver enzymes	ALT, AST, ALP, total bilirubin, direct bilirubin, GGT, lipase
Cholestatic	ALP, bilirubin >> AST, ALT
Hepatocellular	AST, ALT >> ALP/bilirubin
Infiltrative	ALP, GGT >> bilirubin, AST, ALT
Hyperbilirubinemia	High bilirubin only AST/ALT > 2 suggest alcohol
Ammonia	If hepatoencephalopathic
Chronic liver disease workup	ANA, ANCA, ceruloplasmin, TSH, HBsAg, HBeAg, anti-HBs, anti-HBc, anti-HBe, quantitative immunoglobulins, ferritin, Fe, TIBC, alpha-1-antitrypsin, ADP, creatine kinase, haptoglobin, peripheral smear
Additional	US, CT, ERCP

Case 3: Jaundice

A 40-year-old woman presents with jaundice. Please take a history.

Time: 5 minutes

History

HISTORY OF PRESENT ILLNESS

How long have you been jaundiced?
Do you have any of the following symptoms?

- nausea or vomiting
- feeling itchy
- abdominal pain
- fever
- recent weight loss

What color are your stools and urine?

PAST MEDICAL HISTORY

Do you have a history pancreatitis/ERCP, cholecystitis, or liver disease?

Have you ever had blood transfusions?

What medications do you take (Tylenol, antibiotics)?

Is there anyone in your family with liver disease?

What is your sexual orientation?

Have you traveled recently? Where?

Have you had contact with people who have hepatitis or jaundice?

Have you ever used IV drugs?

Do you have a history of abusing ethanol?

Does your work expose you to chemicals harmful to the liver (arsenic, carbon tetrachloride, or vinyl chloride)?

Case 4: Asthma

A person with asthma comes to your office because she has had a cough for the past 2 weeks. Please take a focused history.

Time: 5 minutes

History

HISTORY OF PRESENT ILLNESS

When were you diagnosed with asthma?

What triggers an attack (e.g., exercise, cold, pets)?

Are you a cougher or a wheezer? Do you cough or wheeze at night?

How does your asthma affect your daily activity?

Would you say your asthma is generally well controlled? Poorly controlled?

Are you on any regular medications for asthma?

Do you use salbutamol or other short-acting puffers more than 3 times a week?

Have you been instructed on how to use puffers?

PAST MEDICAL HISTORY

What other medications do you take (beta-blockers, thiazides)?

Do you have allergies?

Have you ever been hospitalized for asthma (intubated, ICU)?

Do you have any family members with asthma?

How old are you?

What do you do for a living?

Does anybody smoke at home?

Do you have any pets at home?

Case 5: Aortic stenosis

A 60-year-old man visits your office because he is worried about an aortic stenosis that was found by his family doctor, although he is currently asymptomatic. Please discuss condition management with the patient.

Time: 10 minutes

Management

Asymptomatic patients:

- have excellent survival (near normal)
- need close follow up and serial echocardiograms if symptoms develop

Counsel the patient about:

- avoiding heavy exertion
- avoiding nitrates/vasodilators
- risk of infectious endocarditis and the need for antibiotic prophylaxis
- risk and symptoms of CHF

ADDITIONAL INFORMATION FOR SYMPTOMATIC PATIENTS

Symptomatic patients have the following risks: ventricular fibrillation, left ventricular failure, and complete heart block.

Long-term prognosis:

- Surgery may be required.
- Patients usually die within 5 years of the onset of syncope, 3 years after onset of angina, and less than 2 years after onset of congestive heart failure/dyspnea.

Case 6: Renal failure

A 48-year-old woman has a critically high creatinine level. Please take a history, do a physical exam, and provide a differential diagnosis and key initial investigations.

Time: 10 minutes

History

Questions should first seek to distinguish chronic from acute renal failure. Depending on that outcome, questions should then target the symptoms of chronic or acute renal failure.

HISTORY OF PRESENT ILLNESS

When were you aware of the elevation of creatine?

Has your kidney function been normal until now?

Do you feel fatigued? What is the fatigue like (e.g., decreased overall energy, decreased exercise tolerance, shortness of breath on exertion)?

Have you had any recent medical imaging with contrast?

Are you experiencing any of the following symptoms? (See breakdown that follows.)

SYMPTOM	SYMPTOM CATEGORY
Retention of water or weight gain (edema), nocturnal muscle cramping, joint effusion	Musculoskeletal
Confusion, inability to concentrate, restless leg syndrome, neuropathy	CNS
Hypertension, congestive heart failure, retinopathy	Cardiovascular
Shortness of breath	Respiratory
Nausea and vomiting, anorexia, constipation, diarrhea	GI
Rash, petechiae, purpura, changes in pigmentation	Dermatological
Hyperlipidemia, menstrual irregularity, low sex drive	Endocrine
Anemia, bleeding, immune compromise	Hematological

PAST MEDICAL HISTORY

Have you had any of the following?

- chronic renal disease
- hypertension
- type 2 diabetes
- SLE
- vasculitides
- hepatitis B or C virus

- recent or recurrent throat infections with group A *Streptococcus*
- malignancy (multiple myeloma)
- voiding difficulties (decrease in stream, dripping, hesitancy, frequency)
- recent or frequent fractures

What medications do you take? For how long?

Has anyone in your family had kidney disease or vasculitis?

FOCUSED QUESTIONS: CHRONIC RENAL FAILURE

Are you experiencing any of the following symptoms? (See breakdown that follows.)

SYMPTOM	POSSIBLE ETIOLOGY
Orthopnea, increased salt intake	Volume overload
Pallor, angina	Anemia (may also involve shortness of breath on exertion)
Malaise, weakness, nausea and vomiting, itchiness (pruritus), yellow skin color	Uremia

Have you had any problems with pregnancies?

FOCUSED QUESTIONS: ACUTE RENAL FAILURE, PRERENAL ORIGIN

Do any of the following conditions or factors apply to you? (See breakdown that follows.)

CONDITION/FACTOR	POSSIBLE ETIOLOGY
Decreased oral intake, high urine production (diuretics, osmotic), sweating, acute bleeding	True decreased intravascular volume
Cirrhosis, malnutrition, severe illness/hospitalization, congestive heart failure, cancer	Decreased effective circulating volume-decreased albumin
Chronic hypertension	Renal artery stenosis and decreased cardiac output to kidney
Use of ACE inhibitors, ARBs, tacrolimus, cocaine, NSAIDs	Decreased cardiac output to kidney

FOCUSED QUESTIONS: ACUTE RENAL FAILURE, RENAL ORIGIN

Do any of the following conditions or factors apply to you? (See breakdown that follows.)

CONDITION/FACTOR	POSSIBLE ETIOLOGY
Hematuria, hemoptysis	Goodpasture syndrome
Recent URTI (group A *Streptococcus*) infection	Glomerular

(Continued)

CONDITION/FACTOR	POSSIBLE ETIOLOGY
Recent use of contrast dye, antibiotics	Tubular toxicity
History of myeloma, gout, hypotension, rhabdomyolysis	
Chronic hypertension, history of emboli or small hemorrhages on skin (petechiae)	Vascular
Use of proton pump inhibitors (PPIs), NSAIDs, sulfonamides, diuretics, vancomycin, rifampin	Interstitial nephritis
Costovertebral angle pain, dysuria, urinary frequency, fever	

FOCUSED QUESTIONS: ACUTE RENAL FAILURE, POSTRENAL ORIGIN

Do any of the following conditions or factors apply to you? (See breakdown that follows.)

CONDITION/FACTOR	POSSIBLE ETIOLOGY
Abdominal pain, hematuria	Stone
Pelvic discomfort, pregnancy (for males: prostate disorders)	Obstruction (may also involve voiding difficulties)
Incontinence, trauma, neurological disease	Neurogenic bladder

Physical exam

CATEGORY TO ASSESS	FINDINGS TO NOTE IF PRESENT
Vitals	HTN
General condition	Uremic fetor, loss of consciousness
CNS	Flapping tremor, mental clouding (uremic encephalopathy)
Cardiovascular symptom	Distant heart sounds (pericardial effusion), pericardial rub, elevated venous pressure, pedal edema
Respiration	Kussmaul respiration, dullness to percussion, decreased breath sounds (pleural effusion)
Abdomen	Renal mass, large bladder
Skin	Sallow complexion, pallor, anemia (normocytic normochromic), ecchymoses, excoriation (pruritus), hyperpigmentation
Other	Signs of infection (impaired cellular immunity)

Investigations

Recommend, as appropriate:

- urinalysis, 24 h urine, Cr, Cr clearance, BUN
- CBC, electrolytes, LFTs, ABG
- kidney-ureter-bladder (KUB) X-ray
- IVP
- renal scan
- US, CT, MRI
- cystoscopy, renal biopsy

Differential diagnosis

See Table 4.

Table 4. DIFFERENTIAL DIAGNOSIS OF RENAL FAILURE

ETIOLOGY	EXAMPLES
Prerenal origin	
Volume depletion	Hemorrhage, gastrointestinal loss, inadequate intake, polyuria, sweating
Reduced effective circulating volume (third-spacing)	Cirrhosis, malnutrition, CHF, protein-losing enteropathy, cancer
Decreased cardiac output	CHF, renal artery stenosis, renal vein thrombosis, cocaine, ACE inhibitors, ARB, sepsis, shock
Renal origin	
Acute tubular necrosis	Ischemia secondary to hemorrhage, hypotension, surgery, burns
Tubular toxicity	Radio contrast, rhabdomyolysis, hemolysis, tumor lysis, myeloma
Infection	Glomerular nephritis, pyelonephritis
Tubulointerstitial disease	NSAIDs, ACE inhibitors, sulfa drugs, proton pump inhibitors (PPIs)
Infiltration	Sarcoidosis, malignancy
Vascular	HTN (chronic or malignant), emboli, scleroderma, vasculitis, HUS/TTP
Chronic kidney disease	Chronic glomerular nephritis, polycystic kidney disease
Postrenal origin	
Ureter obstruction	Blood clots, stones, tumors, papillary necrosis, pregnancy (pressing on ureter)
Urethral obstruction	Strictures, tumor
Prostate	BPH, cancer, prostatitis
Bladder	Cancer, stone, neurogenic

Case 7: Diabetes counseling

A patient newly diagnosed with diabetes comes to you for advice on how to manage her condition.

Time: 5 minutes

History

Take a history to understand the patient's condition before you counsel her, and to determine if the patient has type 1 or type 2 diabetes.

HISTORY OF PRESENT ILLNESS

When did you first find out you had diabetes?

Do you have type 1 or type 2 diabetes?

How old were you when you began experiencing symptoms?

What blood glucose level did you have when you were diagnosed?

Do you experience any of the following?

- excessive thirst, urination, or appetite
- incontinence
- dizziness on standing (orthostatic hypotension)
- early satiety (gastroparesis)
- constipation or diarrhea
- numbness or tingling in your feet
- ulcers on your feet
  - if yes, ask about foot-care routines
- male patients: erectile dysfunction

What do you eat each day?

Are you experiencing changes in your weight?

What exercise do you do? How much, how frequent, for how long?

PAST MEDICAL HISTORY

Has your diabetes ever caused you to lose consciousness or become seriously ill (e.g., diabetic ketoacidosis, hypo-/hyperglycemia)?

Have you been diagnosed with any of the following conditions?

- cardiac conditions (e.g., hypertension, dyslipidemia, myocardial infarction/vascular disease)
- vascular conditions (e.g., claudication, ulcers, dermopathy, infection)

- eye conditions (e.g., retinal hemorrhages, diabetic retinopathy)
  - check date of last ophthalmology assessment
- kidney conditions (e.g., proteinuria, chronic renal disease, diabetic nephropathy)
  - check date and results of last urinalysis
- neuropathy

Do you take insulin? Do you take other medications for diabetes or for other conditions?

Have you ever been hospitalized? What for?

Do other members of your family have diabetes? What kind?

Do you drink or smoke?

Management

Address the patient's specific questions. Begin by asking, "What questions do you have?"

Remember to approach type 1 and type 2 diabetes differently. Type 1 diabetes is an autoimmune disease that classically presents in children; is associated with weight loss, polyuria, and polydipsia; is treated with insulin; and can cause diabetic ketoacidosis if inadequately treated. Type 2 diabetes is associated with insulin resistance, classically presents in overweight individuals, and does not cause diabetic ketoacidosis.

Let the patient know that the complications of diabetes (both type 1 and type 2) include atherosclerosis, nephropathy, retinopathy, neuropathy, and infection. Explain that studies show maintaining glucose levels close to normal can significantly reduce the risk of these complications.

DIET

Counsel the patient to:

- Divide the food they eat in a day into more meals of smaller quantity, such as 3 meals and 3 snacks.
- Avoid simple sugars, saturated fat, and excess salt. Eat regular meals with higher fiber and complex carbohydrates. Aim for meals that are about 50% carbohydrate, 30% fat, and 20% protein. Avoid alcohol.

If the patient has type 2 diabetes, explain that type 2 diabetes can be improved by achieving ideal body weight. The goal is gradual sustained weight reduction of approximately 0.5 to 1 kg/wk (1 to 2 lb/wk).

EXERCISE

Explain that exercise has benefits for people with diabetes: it depletes muscle glycogen and overcomes insulin resistance.

Counsel the patient to:

- Start with light activity, such as walking 4 to 6 times per week for 10 to 30 minutes, achieving 70% to 80% of maximum heart rate.
- Have a stress test before beginning routine rigorous exercise.

Counsel on the patient on controlling other cardiovascular risk factors (e.g., smoking cessation).

MEDICATION AND MONITORING

Oral medications:

- If HbA1C < 9.0, administer metformin.
- If HbA1C > 9.0, administer metformin with another agent from another class or insulin.
- If symptomatic hyperglycemia with metabolic decompensation, administer insulin.

Insulin:

- It is indicated for all type 1 diabetes and decompensated type 2 diabetes.
- Patients should store it in the fridge, draw it accurately, and rotate their injection sites.
- When patients begin taking it, they have several options:
  o Option 1: calculate the dose as 0.5 U/kg (0.2 U/lb).
    - Morning: take two-thirds of the dose (as one-third rapid and two-thirds long-acting).
    - Evening: take one-third of the dose (as half rapid before supper and half NPH before bed).
  o Option 2: start with a 10–15 U dose and increase it by 1–2 U/d until they have good control.
  o Option 3: use a premixed insulin, which they take twice a day.
- Patients should continue insulin even if they feel sick, since their insulin resistance may increase when they are sick.

Counsel the patient about hypoglycemia:

- signs: tremor, palpitation, sweating (autonomic); fatigue, confusion (neurologic)
- what to do: have a syringe of glucagon ready

Counsel the patient about monitoring:

- HbA1C, serum glucose, urinalysis, blood urea nitrogen (BUN), Cr, plasma lipids, ECG, ophthalmology
- blood sugar targets: HbA1C < 7.0, fasting glucose 4.0–7.0, and 2 hours after a meal 5.0–7.0

Case 8: Diabetic ketoacidosis

A patient presents with diabetic ketoacidosis (DKA). Please obtain a focused history, do a physical exam, recommend investigations, and initiate appropriate management.

Time: 10 minutes

History

HISTORY OF PRESENT ILLNESS

When were you diagnosed with diabetes?

How do you control your blood sugars?

What is the cause of the current situation (infections, ischemia, trauma, stopped medications, dehydration)?

How do you feel now?

Do you have any of the following symptoms?

- headache
- shortness of breath
- nausea and vomiting
- dizziness
- confusion

Physical exam

Assess:

- vitals
- LOC
- general appearance: Kussmaul breathing, smell (fruity/acetone)
- signs of dehydration (dry skin/mucous membranes, poor turgor)
- signs of infection/trauma
- signs of insulin injection and DM complications

Investigations

INVESTIGATION CATEGORY	DETAILS
General chemistry	CBC, electrolytes, glucose, ketones, ABG, urinalysis, ECG
Diabetic ketoacidosis diagnosis	Elevated blood glucose; increased serum acetoacetate, acetone, and hydroxybutyrate metabolic acidosis (low serum bicarbonate and low blood pH); increased anion gap

Management

Ensure ABCs:

- Establish 2 large bore IVs.
- Start oxygen.
- Start monitors for vital signs.

Rehydration: administer 1 L/h NS for first 2 h (patient will have a fluid deficit of 6–10 L).

Insulin IV: push 10 U, then 10 U/h.

ABG: repeat to monitor K$^+$ levels and anion gap for ketones.

In case of cerebral edema: administer mannitol.

MANAGEMENT IN FIRST HOUR

Volume replacement: administer a total 3–5 L with NS.

Insulin bolus: administer 0.15 U/kg (0.065 U/lb), then sliding scale infusion.

On patient's first urination: add 20 mEq KCl to NS.

Monitor hourly glucose, K, electrolytes (anion gap), and urine output.

Monitor ketosis with anion gap.

Case 9: Hypertension

A 50-year-old university professor presents with a blood pressure reading of 160/98. He has undergone tests for HTN and had a physical examination, all of which had normal results. Please take a focused history and discuss with the patient how to manage his condition.

Time: 5 minutes

History

In this case, history taking should have the following goals: to confirm the diagnosis, rule out secondary causes and exogenous causes, and to screen for cardiovascular risk factors.

HISTORY OF PRESENT ILLNESS

When did you notice your blood pressure was high? How high was it?

Was it treated? How did that go?

When was your last normal blood pressure reading?

Have you been experiencing any of the following symptoms?

- chest pain
- shortness of breath
- leg discomfort, difficulty walking
- vision changes
- changes in your body (voice, hair, bruising, skin color, weight loss)
- episodes of sweating profusely, palpitations, or headache

Have you had any recent stresses in your life?

When was the last time your cholesterol was checked?

PAST MEDICAL HISTORY

Have you ever had a heart attack or stroke?

Have you been diagnosed with any of the following?

- aortic dissection
- pulmonary edema
- diabetes
- kidney disease

Do you snore?

Do you have a history of early morning headaches and daytime somnolence?

Are you on any medications (amphetamine, oral contraceptive, licorice, thyroid hormone)?

Does anyone in your family have high blood pressure?

What is your diet like?

What do you do for exercise? How often? How long?

Do you smoke, drink, or use recreational drugs?

Management

Depending on the information from the history, counsel the patient to take the following steps:

- Stop smoking.
- Restrict salt intake.
- Restrict alcohol consumption.
- Reduce and control weight (if over 115% of ideal body weight).
- Get regular aerobic exercise.
- Modify life circumstances to reduce stress.

If these steps do not reduce the patient's blood pressure in the next 3 to 6 months, then a blood pressure medication is necessary.

Case 10: Anemia

A young woman's routine physical examination for employment has shown abnormal hemoglobin and reticulocyte counts. Please take a history.

Time: 5 minutes

History

HISTORY OF PRESENT ILLNESS

Have you had abnormal results for hemoglobin and reticulocyte counts before?

When was the first time?

Are you experiencing any of the following?

- shortness of breath on exertion
- palpitations, headache, angina, or increasing fatigue

What are your stools like (dark/tarry, bloody, diarrhea)?

PAST MEDICAL HISTORY

Do you have frequent nosebleeds?

Do you have a history of oral, respiratory, gastrointestinal, or genitourinary bleeding?

Do you have a history of any of the following?

- dyspepsia
- gastroesophageal reflux disease
- peptic ulcers
- chronic disease of the liver, kidney, or bowel

Do any of the following symptoms or factors apply to you? (See breakdown that follows.)

SYMPTOM/FACTOR	POSSIBLE ETIOLOGY
Use of ASA, NSAIDs, blood thinners	Occult blood loss
Vegetarian diet, insufficient diet (due to financial difficulties, time, interest)	Iron deficiency
Fever, night sweats, adenopathy, weight change	Malignancy
Mediterranean/Asian origins	Genetic
Gastric surgery, inflammatory bowel disease, hypothyroidism, raw fish intake, celiac disease	B_{12} deficiency
Vitiligo, glossitis, neuropsychiatric symptoms	
Alcohol abuse, poor nutrition, pregnancy, blood dyscrasia, celiac disease, psoriasis, anticonvulsant use, or antimetabolite therapy	Folate deficiency
Itchiness, dark brown urine	Hemolysis

Are any members of your family anemic?

How old were you when you had your first period?

How long is your usual cycle? How many days of bleeding are usual for you? How many pads or tampons do you usually use per day? Are there clots?

Has there been any change in your cycle?

Case 11: Megaloblastic anemia

A 69-year-old man is experiencing fatigue, dizziness, and an unsteady gait. Lab results show the following: mean corpuscular volume (MCV) 120, hemoglobin (Hb) 90, white blood count 3.4. Please take a history, perform a focused physical exam, and determine what further investigations may be required.

Time: 10 minutes

History

The patient's high MCV and low Hb suggest megaloblastic anemia. History taking should focus on distinguishing this cause from other possible causes of increased MCV (e.g., medications, myelodysplastic syndromes).

HISTORY OF PRESENT ILLNESS

When did you begin experiencing your symptoms (fatigue, dizziness, unsteady gait)?

Do you have diarrhea?

Have you experienced any of the following?

- increased bleeding (mouth, nose)
- bruising

PAST MEDICAL HISTORY

What medications do you take (folate inhibitors, antiretroviral drugs)?

Do you have a history of ethanol abuse?

Physical exam

The physical exam should focus on signs of megaloblastic anemia and myelodysplastic syndromes.

Check for:

- coordination with eyes open versus eyes closed
- purpura
- splenomegaly
- hepatomegaly

Investigations

INVESTIGATION CATEGORY	DETAILS
Megaloblastic anemia	Schiller test, bone marrow analysis, B_{12} level, blood smear
Myelodysplastic syndromes	CBC, peripheral blood smear, bone marrow examination

Case 12: Angina and acute MI

A 55-year-old man presents with crushing retrosternal chest pain. His blood pressure is 110/80, and his heart rate is 180 and irregular. Please take a focused history, perform a physical exam, interpret the patient's ECG, and initiate appropriate management.

Time: 10 minutes

History

The history should first focus on the patient's acute pain. Mnemonics may help:

- **OLD CARS**: **o**nset, **l**ocations, **d**uration, **c**haracter, **a**ssociated symptoms, **r**adiation, **s**everity (shown below)
- **OPQRST**: **o**nset, **p**recipitating, **q**uantity, **r**elieving, **s**everity, **t**iming

Because of the acute nature of the case, the history should then assess: risks posed by administering streptokinase, followed by the patient's risk for cardiovascular events and thromboembolism.

While taking the history, watch for easily visible signs such as dyspnea, hand warmth, sweating, peripheral cyanosis, clubbing, nail splinter hemorrhages, and jugular venous pressure.

HISTORY OF PRESENT ILLNESS (MNEMONIC: OLD CARS)

ONSET

When did your symptoms begin?

Did the symptoms come on suddenly or gradually?

What were you doing when the symptoms began?

LOCATION

Can you point to the place that hurts the most?

DURATION

How long does the pain usually last? Minutes, hours?

Have you experienced any changes in the duration lately?

How frequently are you having pain? Any changes in frequency of the pain?

Does the pain go away when you rest? How long does it take?

CHARACTER

What is the pain like (e.g., cutting, aching, burning, "heaviness")?

Have you ever had any similar pain?

Do you get pain in your chest on exertion?

Have you experienced symptoms while at rest?

Does it get worse with cold air or after a big meal?

How many blocks you can walk without symptoms (chest pain)?

ASSOCIATED SYMPTOMS

Do any of the following symptoms/factors apply to you?

- shortness of breath
- nausea and vomiting
- fever
- recent weight loss
- calf pain
- palpitations
- lightheadedness, muscular weakness, or feeling faint
- heartburn, acid reflux, or difficulty swallowing
- rash (e.g., shingles)
- cough
- strained muscles
- stress in your life

RADIATION

Does the pain stay in the chest or does it radiate to the arm, back, or shoulder?

SEVERITY

How severe is the pain?

FOCUSED QUESTIONS: STREPTOKINASE

Have you been treated with streptokinase?

Do you have any drug allergies?

FOCUSED QUESTIONS: CARDIOVASCULAR SYSTEM

Have you been diagnosed with any of the following?

- type 2 diabetes
- hypertension
- high cholesterol (dyslipidemia)

Male patients younger than 45, female patients older than 55:

- Has anyone in your family had a heart attack?

Do you smoke?

FOCUSED QUESTIONS: THROMBOEMBOLISM

Have you been diagnosed with chronic venous insufficiency?

Have you had surgery recently?

Have you been immobilized recently?

Have you recently been inactive (e.g., sitting or lying down for a prolonged period of time)?

Have you had a leg injury or any swelling in your legs?

Have you had pain in your lungs (pleuritic chest pain)?

Female patients:

- Do you take heparin or birth control pills?
- When was your last menstrual period?
- Are you pregnant?

Physical exam

Place the patient in a comfortable position:

- pulmonary edema: sitting up
- syncope, hypovolemia, or pulmonary embolism: lying down

CATEGORY TO ASSESS	DETAILS
Vitals	BP (both arms, supine and upright)
	• orthostatic hypotension
	° SBP drop over 20
	° DBP drop over 10
	• pulse: pulse pressure, pulsus alternans, pulsus paradoxus drop over 10 during inspiration
	• heart rate, respiration rate, O_2 saturation
Head and neck	Dyspnea, cyanosis, diaphoresis, jugular venous pressure
Arterial pulse	Rate, rhythm, amplitude, contour, bruit
Chest	Inspection: precordial apex beat, heaves, lifts, breathing pattern, any abnormal pulsation
	Palpation: apex beat (size and character), vibrations or thrills
	Percussion: heart size
	Heart auscultation:
	• regularity
	• murmur (timing, duration, rate, pitch, intensity, pattern, quality, location, radiation, relation to respiration)
	• splitting or extra sounds
	• opening snap, clicks, pericardial rubs
	• carotid artery (radiating murmur or bruits)

(*Continued*)

CATEGORY TO ASSESS	DETAILS
Chest (continued)	Pulmonary auscultation (both front and back):
	• pleural effusion (heart border)
	• crackles (pulmonary edema)
Abdomen (lie patient flat, if tolerated)	Liver (palpate): hepatomegaly, hepatojugular reflex, aortic aneurysm
	Abdominal aorta (auscultate): renal, iliac, and femoral bruit
Extremities	Pulse: femoral, popliteal, dorsalis pedis, posterior tibialis pulses
	Ankle or sacral edema, bilateral or unilateral

ECG interpretation

The basics of ECG interpretation include:

- rate
- rhythm: P waves; QRS (wide or narrow); P and QRS relation; regularity
- axis: normal positive QRS in I and II
- waves and segments
- hypertrophy and chamber enlargement
- ischemia and infarction
- miscellaneous: hyper/hypokalemia, hyper/hypocalcemia, pericarditis, digoxin toxicity

Management of the MI patient

Ensure ABCs:

- Stabilize.
- Establish IV.
- Start oxygen to keep saturation over 95%.
- Start monitors: cardiac, 12-lead ECG (have previous ECG to compare).

Administer:

- ASA 325 mg to chew
- nitroglycerin sublingual q5min × 3/nitropatch/nitroglycerin drip (contraindicated with sildenafil or suspected right ventricular infarct)
- morphine 2–5 mg IV
- anticoagulant: low molecular weight heparin
- thrombolytics
- beta-blocker
- lipid control
- blood pressure support

Initiate investigations:

- troponin (6 h after onset and q6h × 2), CBC, electrolytes, Cr, urea, CXR

Assess whether to consult cardiology or coronary care unit.

Assess patient for percutaneous coronary intervention (PCI):

- thrombolysis contraindicated
- patient presents more than 12 hours post onset with continued pain, or has had previous coronary artery bypass graft surgery (CABG), or develops shock

Assess patient for CABG:

- left main disease greater than 50%
- 2-vessel disease (1 must be left anterior descending), or diffuse 3-vessel disease

Case 13: Pneumonia, pleurisy

A patient presents with pneumonia and coughing. Perform a physical exam, interpret the patient's X-ray, and recommend appropriate management.

Time: 10 minutes

History

The history should focus on distinguishing bacterial from nonbacterial etiology, and rule out pulmonary embolism.

While taking the history, watch for respiratory distress (nasal flare, pursed lip breathing, using of accessory muscles, in-drawing), and for clues such as oxygen supplementation and sputum-laden tissues.

During the history, practice infection control.

HISTORY OF PRESENT ILLNESS

When did you come down with pneumonia?

Are you experiencing any of the following symptoms?

- shortness of breath (when lying down, at night)
- exercise intolerance
- fever

- chest pain (e.g., when you breathe)
- loss of consciousness
- diarrhea, confusion, bradycardia

Have you had a recent respiratory infection?

Have you modified any of your usual activities because you feel sick?

What is your cough like (productive, wheezy, nocturnal, position dependent)?

Have you experienced a change in cough pattern?

What are you coughing up (green, pink, frothy, red current jelly–like, containing blood or pus)?

Do you drink? Were you drunk the day before?

Do you have a head trauma or neurological disorder?

PAST MEDICAL HISTORY

Have you had a similar episode before?

Have you ever been diagnosed with any of the following?

- asthma
- eczema
- TB
- respiratory infection
- chronic lung disease
- HIV
- PCP (*Pneumocystis jiroveci* pneumonia)
- CMV (cytomegalic virus)
- mycobacterium infection

Do you have allergies?

Does your family have a history of allergies, eczema, or asthma?

What do you do for a living?

Do you smoke?

Do you have pets at home?

Have you traveled recently? Where?

Have you been in contact with anyone who has TB?

Physical exam

During the physical exam, it is crucial to practice infection control.

CATEGORY TO ASSESS	DETAILS
Vitals	Temperature, respiration rate, O_2 saturation
General condition	Chills/rigors, LOC, posture, diaphoresis, cyanosis
Respiratory system	Hands: clubbing, cyanosis (central, peripheral), nicotine stain CO_2 retention: tremor, headache, warm extremities, pounding pulse
	Jugular venous pressure (cor pulmonale), CHF
	Supraclavicular lymph node
	Inspection (chest):
	• pattern of breathing, rate, rhythm, depth
	• chest wall deformity and inequality of movement: barrel chest, kyphosis, scoliosis, pectus excavatum, flail chest, retractions and contractions
	Palpation: displacement of trachea; chest wall tenderness, vocal fremitus; crepitus, pericardial pulsation; chest expansion
	Percussion: dullness, hyperresonance, diaphragmatic excursion
	Auscultation (chest):
	• Listen for overt adventitious sounds (e.g., wheezes, vocal resonance, whispering pectoriloquy, decreased breath sounds, pleural friction rub, transmitted sound).
	• If appropriate, measure flow rate.
	• During heart auscultation, listen for S3 gallop (CHF).

Chest X-ray interpretation (posterior/anterior and lateral)

See Table 5.

Table 5. INTERPRETING X-RAYS FOR PNEUMONIA (PATCHY, DIFFUSE INFILTRATE)

INFILTRATE CATEGORY	ETIOLOGY
Atypical	Legionella, Mycoplasma, viral, aspiration, Pneumocystis jiroveci pneumonia
Segmental or lobar	Pneumococcal infection
Parapneumonic effusion	Complications, abscess, emphysema, pneumothorax

Management

Administer medication as appropriate (see Table 6).

Table 6. MEDICATION INDICATED FOR TYPES OF PNEUMONIA

CONDITION	MEDICATION (SUBJECT TO LOCAL ANTIBIOGRAMS)
Community acquired typical pneumonia	Levofloxacin 500 mg po daily × 6 d
Community acquired atypical pneumonia	Azithromycin 500 mg po × 1d, then 250 mg × 4 d
Aspiration pneumonia	Ceftriaxone 1g IV q24h and metronidazole 500 mg IV ql2h
Nursing home or nosocomial pneumonia	Ceftriaxone 1g IV/IM ql2h or vancomycin
If at risk of aspiration	Metronidazole 500 mg tid plus cefotaxime 1–2 g q8h or imipenem 500 mg IV 16 h

Counsel the patient to:

- Drink adequate fluids.
- Take their temperature every evening.
- Avoid overuse of cough suppressants, as coughing helps clear the airway. Use only at night for sleep.
- Stop smoking.
- Watch for evidence of worsening symptoms: unremitting fever, drowsiness, shortness of breath (dyspnea), and blue coloration at base of fingernails, on tongue, or around lips (cyanosis).
- Stop the spread of their illness to others (e.g., stay home while sick, avoid preparing food for others).

Case 14: Chest pain and respiratory distress

A patient presents with dyspnea and chest pain. Please perform a physical exam, provide a differential diagnosis, and recommend appropriate investigations.

Time: 10 minutes

Physical exam

CATEGORY TO ASSESS	DETAILS
Vitals	Temperature, respiration rate, O_2 saturation
General condition	LOC
Cardiovascular system	S1, S2, jugular venous pressure, carotid pulse, bruits
Respiratory system	Inspection: • pattern of breathing, rate, rhythm, depth • chest wall deformity and inequality of movement: barrel chest, kyphosis, scoliosis, pectus excavatum, flail chest, retractions and contractions Palpation: displacement of trachea; chest wall tenderness, vocal fremitus; crepitus, pericardial pulsation; chest expansion Percussion: dullness, hyperresonance, diaphragmatic excursion Auscultation: • Listen for overt adventitious sounds (e.g., wheezes, vocal resonance, whispering pectoriloquy, decreased breath sounds, pleural friction rub, transmitted sound). • If appropriate, measure flow rate. • During heart auscultation, listen for S3 gallop (CHF).
Abdomen	Palpation: tenderness, mass especially AAA, liver, spleen Auscultation: bowel sounds and bruit
Legs	Edema, phlebitis, vascular insufficiency, signs of deep vein thrombosis, calf circumference (measure both sides), peripheral pulses
Cervical and thoracic spine	Neurological signs
Skin	Cyanosis, herpetic rash, pallor, jaundice, xanthomata, anemia

Differential diagnosis

See Table 7.

Table 7. DIFFERENTIAL DIAGNOSIS OF CHEST PAIN

CATEGORY	POSSIBLE ETIOLOGY
Chest wall	Muscle spasm, strain, Tietze disease, rib fracture, cervical/thoracic spine/nerve root compression, herpes, metastatic cancer
Cardiac	Ischemia pericarditis, tamponade
Lung and pleural	Pneumothorax, pulmonary embolus, pneumonia, bronchospasm
GI	Reflux, spasm, ulcer, cholecystitis, pancreatitis
Psychogenic	Anxiety, depression, malingering
Fat embolus	Recent major fracture

Investigations

INVESTIGATION CATEGORY	DETAILS
Chemistry	Cardiac enzymes, ABG
Imaging	ECG, CXR, ventilation-perfusion (V/Q) scan

Case 15: Pulmonary embolism and anticoagulant use

A patient with a pulmonary embolism wants advice about anticoagulant use. Please take a history and discuss anticoagulant management with the patient.

Time: 5 minutes

History

The history needs to focus first on the present problem: the patient's concerns about anticoagulant use. It then needs to assess complications the patient may have with anticoagulant use.

HISTORY OF PRESENT ILLNESS

When was the anticoagulant prescribed?

Are you taking the medication? If not, why?

Are you experiencing any side effects?

Do any of the following factors or conditions apply to you?

- pregnancy (current or planned)
- recent childbirth

- heavy or unusual menstrual bleeding
- planned or recent insertion of an IUD
- fall, blows to the body/head
- fever lasting for more than a couple of days
- planned or recent surgery (medical, dental)
- severe or continuing diarrhea
- recent spinal anesthesia
- planned or recent radiation treatment

PAST MEDICAL HISTORY

Do you have any allergies (sulfates/preservatives in food, medications)?

Are you on a special diet (low salt/sugar)?

How old are you?

Management

Explain the nature of anticoagulants:

- They decrease the clotting ability of the blood and therefore prevent harmful clots from forming in the blood vessels.
- They are sometimes called blood thinners, but they don't actually thin the blood.
- They do not dissolve clots that have already formed, but prevent clots from becoming larger and causing more serious problems.

Counsel the patient about what to do while on the anticoagulant:

- Eat a normal, balanced diet.
- See you before beginning any new medications.
- See you if any new medical problems develop.
- Avoid pregnancy (anticoagulants may cause birth defects).
- Inform relevant medical doctors, dentists, and pharmacists about the medication, or carry medical alert identification.
- Avoid injuries (sports, kitchen). If injury occurs, report to a health center as serious internal bleeding may occur.
- Store medication out of reach of children and away from heat or direct light or moisture. Discard outdated medication

Counsel the patient about how to take the medication:

- Take only as directed.
- Missed dose: take as soon as possible. If missed for a day, don't take on the next day: doubling the dose may cause bleeding.

- Use caution for 2 to 3 weeks after stopping medication.
- Blood tests (INR): daily for 5 days, then every 3 days for 2 weeks, and then weekly.

Case 16: Paroxysmal atrial tachycardia

A 60-year-old woman presents with paroxysmal atrial tachycardia while on digoxin. Her pulse is irregular on examination. She is concerned about taking digoxin, particularly because she plans to vacation in Florida soon. Please take a history and discuss the management of the patient's condition with digoxin.

Time: 5 minutes

History

HISTORY OF PRESENT ILLNESS

When were you diagnosed with paroxysmal atrial tachycardia?

What were your symptoms at the time?

Does anything trigger an attack?

When does it happen (e.g., at rest, with activity, after a meal)?

Can you do anything to stop the attack?

What did you do when you had an attack?

What medications do you take for your condition (digoxin, warfarin, diltiazem, ASA, beta-blockers)?

When did you start these medications? What dosages do you take? Are you taking them as prescribed?

Do you have any of the following symptoms now?
- shortness of breath
- palpitations
- fatigue
- leg swelling

Do these symptoms get worse when you exercise?

PAST MEDICAL HISTORY

Have you ever been diagnosed with any of the following conditions?
- myocardial infarction
- angina
- hypertension

- congestive heart failure
- type 2 diabetes
- high cholesterol
- stroke

Do any of these conditions run in your family?

Other than medications you take for paroxysmal atrial tachycardia, what medications do you take?

Do you drink or smoke?

Management

Begin by asking the patient what she knows about paroxysmal atrial tachycardia and how digoxin works. Ask if she has any particular concerns about digoxin, and address her concerns directly.

As appropriate, review the nature of paroxysmal atrial tachycardia:

- The heart beats too fast and irregularly.
- It doesn't pump blood effectively, which causes symptoms of heart failure: chest pain, shortness of breath, headache, cough, swelling of the feet, etc.
- Blood clots form easily, which cause stroke and peripheral thromboembolism.

As appropriate, review the effects of digoxin:

- It slows the heart down and makes it beat stronger.
- On a therapeutic dose, the side effects are minimal.
- Side effects to watch for include: blurred or yellowed vision, headache, drowsiness, green color blindness, nausea, syncope, etc.

Counsel the patient that:

- It is necessary to control her heart rate.
- Right now, she is not getting enough digoxin.
- It is important to take the prescribed dose.
- She needs to let you know if she goes on any other medications, so that you can monitor drug interaction (especially cimetidine, theophylline, phenobarbital, etc.).

Counsel her on controlling other risk factors (e.g., alcohol use, smoking cessation).

Arrange to recheck her digoxin level after 1 week and adjust the dose as necessary.

Reassure her that the correct dose will control her condition, and reassure her about her vacation in Florida.

Case 17: Hemoptysis, cardiac failure

A 60-year-old man is experiencing hemoptysis and shortness of breath. Please take a history and provide a management strategy.

Time: 5 minutes

History

The patient has 2 presenting conditions (hemoptysis, shortness of breath). The history needs to explore them individually. Note that some of the questions apply to both conditions (chest pain, dizziness, palpitations, diaphoresis, medications), so you only ask them once.

HISTORY OF PRESENT ILLNESS (HEMOPTYSIS)

When did this start?

Did it start suddenly or gradually?

Does it happen chronically (e.g., every winter or spring)?

Where is the bleeding?

- Are you coughing up blood or vomiting blood?
- Do you have a nosebleed or bleeding gums?

What is the sputum like (e.g., bloody, pink, putrid, puss-filled, copious)?

Have you had contact with anyone sick?

Do you have any of the following symptoms?

- chest pain, dizziness, palpitations, excessive sweating, low urine output
- night sweats, weight loss
- other unusual bleeding (e.g., gums, skin bruising)
- blood in your urine
- fever

Have you had TB or recent contact with TB?

Have you been diagnosed with kidney disease?

What medications are you taking (ASA, anticoagulants, antibiotics, NSAIDs, puffers, home oxygen, beta-blockers)?

Have you recently had surgery?

Do any of your family members have similar problems?

Do you smoke? How much a day? How many years?

Have you traveled to TB-endemic areas?

What do you do for a living? Does your occupation expose you to any lung toxins (e.g., asbestos)?

HISTORY OF PRESENT ILLNESS (BREATHLESSNESS)

When did the feeling of breathlessness start?

Is it worse on exertion or lying down?

How well did you tolerate exercise before this symptom?

How many pillows do you sleep on?

Do you cough or wheeze when you are having shortness of breath?

Are you experiencing nausea or vomiting?

Are you experiencing stress in your life?

Management

Ensure ABCs.

Treat underlying disease: coronary artery disease (CAD), HTN, hyperthyroidism, hypothyroidism.

Treat precipitating factors: anemia, fever, pneumonia, pulmonary embolus, exertion, emotion, high dose beta-blocker.

Prescribe:

- salt-restricted diet (2 g/d)
- diuretic (except in case of aortic stenosis)
- ACE inhibitor
- statin
- anticoagulant

If you prescribe digoxin, monitor heart rate, rhythm, and serum K and Mg.

For cardiogenic shock, prescribe a beta-blocker. If the patient has stable atrial fibrillation, amiodarone is the first choice.

Avoid calcium channel blockers.

Case 18: Lymphadenopathy

A young woman presents with night sweats and lymphadenopathy, which comes and goes. Obtain a history, perform a physical exam, provide a differential diagnosis, and recommend investigations.

Time: 10 minutes

History

The history needs to determine how long the patient has experienced inflammation. Think **rule of 7s**:

- 7 days: inflammatory
- 7 months: tumor
- 7 years: congenital

HISTORY OF PRESENT ILLNESS

When did you notice you had enlarged lymph nodes?

Did it happen suddenly or gradually?

Where did it start? Did it spread to other nodes?

Are the enlarged nodes on one side only or both sides?

Have you had contact with anyone sick?

Have you been injured recently?

Do you have any of the following symptoms?

- fever
- pain
- sore throat
- urinary changes
- rash or skin changes
- watery or red eyes
- wheezing or hoarseness (recurrent laryngeal nerve compression of aortopulmonary window)
- cough, shortness of breath, facial swelling (mediastinal nodes)
- swelling in your lower extremities (retroperitoneal nodes)

PAST MEDICAL HISTORY

Do you have a history of any of the following?

- upper respiratory tract infections
- STDs
- exposure to TB

- fatigue, weakness, weight loss, night sweats, abdominal pain, back pain, epigastric pain (Assess for malignancy.)
- loss of appetite
- weight loss
- testicular mass (if male)
- coughing up blood

What medications do you take?

Has anyone in your family been diagnosed with an illness?

How old are you?

What do you do for a living?

Do you smoke or use recreational drugs?

Physical exam

Check:

- general appearance: cachexia, anemia, fever
- vitals
- head and neck: ear, eye, nose, nasopharynx, throat, oral cavity, larynx (especially if upper neck lymphadenopathy)
- lymph node groups: occipital, posterior auricular/mastoid, preauricular/parotid, submandibular, submental, anterior cervical chain, posterior cervical chain, clavicular, subclavicular
- Virchow node: left side suggests GI; right side suggests lung, mediastinum, chest
- thyroid
- breasts and axillary nodes
- abdomen: splenomegaly, inguinal nodes, liver

Describe each lymph node in terms of size, mobility, tenderness, shape, and consistency.

Differential diagnosis

See Table 8.

Table 8. DIFFERENTIAL DIAGNOSIS OF LYMPHADENOPATHY

TYPE	POSSIBLE ETIOLOGY
Infectious	Mononucleosis, URTI, HIV, TB, skin infection
Inflammatory	Sarcoidosis, SLE
Neoplastic	Metastatic tumor, lymphoma (Hodgkin/non-Hodgkin), leukemia

Investigations

INVESTIGATION	REASON
CBC, blood smear	R/O hematological disorder
CXR	R/O nonpalpable lymph nodes, lung mass, evidence of TB or sarcoidosis
Mantoux skin test, sputum culture and stain for acid-fast bacilli	If TB suspected
TSH, free thyroxine (T4), thyroid scan, US, CT, fine needle aspiration (FNA), biopsy	If thyroid cancer suspected
Quadroscopy (larynx, nasopharynx, oropharynx and nasal passages) CT sinuses, FNA, biopsy)	If head and neck cancer suspected
CXR, bronchoscopy	If lung cancer suspected
Air contrast barium swallow, gastroscopy, colonoscopy	If GI cancer suspected
ACE level	If sarcoidosis exacerbation suspected

Case 19: Hilar adenopathy

A 50-year-old woman presents with hilar adenopathy. Please give a differential diagnosis, and recommend and explain blood tests.

Time: 5 minutes

Differential diagnosis

See Table 9.

Table 9. DIFFERENTIAL DIAGNOSIS OF HILAR ADENOPATHY

TYPE	POSSIBLE ETIOLOGY
Neoplastic	Lymphoma, bronchial carcinoma, metastatic tumor
Inflammatory	Sarcoidosis, Churg-Strauss syndrome, amyloidosis, histiocytosis
Infectious	Local infections, TB, HIV, berylliosis

Investigations

INVESTIGATION	REASON
CBC with differential	Leukocytosis (infection), lymphopenia (HIV, sarcoid), increased immature lymphocytes (lymphoma), anemia of chronic disease

(Continued)

INVESTIGATION	REASON
Blood cultures/sputum, acid-fast bacilli	TB
Calcium with albumin	High total protein and hypercalcemia (sarcoidosis), hyperglobulinemia (lymphoma, sarcoidosis)
ACE level	Sarcoidosis
HIV serology	HIV

Case 20: Hypothyroidism

A 40-year-old woman presents with hypothyroidism. Please obtain a history, perform a physical exam, and provide a differential diagnosis.

Time: 10 minutes

History

The history should begin with an assessment of the patient's current condition, and then focus on etiology.

HISTORY OF PRESENT ILLNESS

How do you feel?

Do you find that you are easily fatigued, out of proportion with the activities you do?

Do you feel depressed or suicidal?

Have you noticed any changes in any of the following?

- daily activity
- sleep
- appetite or weight
- frequency of bowel movements
- skin or hair (dry)
- voice (hoarseness)
- menstrual cycle
- vision (blurring, tunnel vision)
- sense of smell
- hearing (loss)

Do you have stiffness or cramping in your muscles?

Do you have swelling in your legs or face?

Do you have numbness or pain in your hands? What relieves it (e.g., shaking, dangling, rubbing)? (Assess for carpal tunnel syndrome.)

FOCUSED QUESTIONS: ETIOLOGY OF HYPOTHYROIDISM

Do any of the following conditions or factors apply to you?

- thyroid enlargement or neck mass
- neck pain
- recent URTI
- pregnant now or recently
- past neck surgery, thyroidectomy, pituitary surgery, or radiation therapy
- taking lithium, iodine, ASA, interferon, thalidomide
- contact with others who have the same problem
- past hyperthyroidism (subacute thyroiditis, postpartum)

Physical exam

CATEGORY	DETAILS
Vitals	Tachycardia/bradycardia, tachypnea, widened pulse pressure
General inspection	Anxiety/somnolence, body habitus, affect, clothing thickness, diaphoresis, thinning hair
Neck	Anterior and lateral view
	Size, goiter, symmetry, erythema
Eyes	Hyperthyroidism:
	• stare/proptosis/ptosis
	• lid lag with downward eye movement
	• widened palpebral fissures
	• chemosis
	• poor convergence
	• exophthalmos
	Hypothyroidism:
	• dry eyes
	• Queen Anne sign
Hands	Brittle nails
	Pemberton sign (thoracic outlet syndrome with raising of hands causes plethora and dilation of cervical veins)
Reflexes	Hyperreflexia, "hung" reflexes

Palpation:

- Examine from anterior and posterior.
- Landmark from cricothyroid cartilage.

- Evaluate everything with and without swallowing (give a glass of water when asking the patient to swallow).
- Evaluate size, consistency, and tenderness over lobes and isthmus.
- Turn head to same side as that palpated to get behind sternocleidomastoid muscle (SCM).
- Palpate nodes.

Auscultation: listen for thyroid bruits.

Differential diagnosis

See Table 10.

Table 10. DIFFERENTIAL DIAGNOSIS OF HYPOTHYROIDISM

TYPE	ETIOLOGY
Primary (95% of cases)	Thyroiditis: Hashimoto, postpartum, subacute
	Iatrogenic: antithyroid drugs (lithium, propylthiouracil, para-aminosalicylic acid, contrast), postradiation, subtotal thyroidectomy
	Iodine deficiency
	Biosynthetic defect
	Infiltration (hemochromatosis, amyloidosis)
Secondary	Pituitary macroadenoma
	Empty sella syndrome
	Infarction
	Sarcoidosis
	Surgery
	Radiation
	Infection
	Infiltration: measure free thyroxine (T4) and other pituitary markers
Tertiary	Hypothalamic

Case 21: Hypercalcemia

A patient presents with elevated serum calcium. Please take a focused history, perform a physical exam, provide a differential diagnosis, and recommend relevant investigations and a plan for management.

Time: 10 minutes

History

HISTORY OF PRESENT ILLNESS

When did you find out you had elevated calcium levels in your blood?

What is the level?

How many tests have you had for it?

Did all the tests show the same level?

When were the tests done?

Do you have any of the following symptoms? (See breakdown that follows.)

SYMPTOM	SYMPTOM CATEGORY
Fatigue, weakness, weight loss, lethargy	General
Constipation, abdominal tenderness/pain (pancreatitis, epigastric pain), loss of appetite, weight loss, nausea, vomiting	GI
Confusion, psychosis, depression, loss of interest in usual activities (lassitude)	CNS
Kidney stones or pain, low or high urine output, frequent urination, excessive thirst	GU
Muscle weakness, bone pain, joint pain	Musculoskeletal
Vision changes or eye pain (band keratopathy)	Other
Cough, breast mass, bone pain, headache	Possible underlying malignancy

PAST MEDICAL HISTORY

Have you been diagnosed with any of the following?

- high blood pressure
- metastatic calcification

How much milk do you drink?

Do you take any of the following? How much?

- antacids
- thiazides
- vitamin D

Has anyone in your family been diagnosed with hypercalcemia?

Physical exam

CATEGORY TO ASSESS	FINDINGS TO NOTE IF PRESENT
Vitals	Elevated BP; orthostatic changes (in cases of dehydration)
Mental status	Confusion, encephalopathy
Signs of malignancy	Cachexia, weight loss, breast/lung/abdominal mass, lymphadenopathy, bony tenderness
HEENT	Parathyroid tumor, band keratopathy, lymphadenopathy (sarcoidosis)
Musculoskeletal system	Bone/muscle weakness, hyporeflexia

Differential diagnosis

Possible etiologies of hypercalcemia include:

- hyperparathyroidism: primary, secondary (renal failure), tertiary
- malignancy: breast, lung (PTHrp), kidney, multiple myeloma
- hyperthyroidism
- Addison disease
- medications: Li, thiazides, vitamin D, calcium
- granulomatous disease
- familial hypocalciuric hypercalcemia
- multiple endocrine neoplasia (MEN) or hypocalciuric hypercalcemia/milk alkali syndrome
- immobilization

Investigations

See Table 11.

Table 11. INVESTIGATIONS FOR HYPERCALCEMIA

SUSPECTED ETIOLOGY	INVESTIGATIONS
Malignancy	Parathyroid hormone (PTH), parathyroid hormone-related protein (PTHrp), electrolytes, Ca^{2+}, phosphate, urine cyclic adenosine monophosphate (cAMP)
Hyperparathyroidism	ALP, bone scan, spinal X-rays (bone mets or subperiosteal bone absorption)

(*Continued*)

Table 11. (*Continued*)

SUSPECTED ETIOLOGY	INVESTIGATIONS
Absorptive hypercalciuria	24 h Ca excretion, serum vitamin D
Multiple myeloma	CBC, ESR, serum protein electrophoresis (SPEP)
Hilar adenopathy, pulmonary findings	CXR
Sarcoidosis	ACE level
Hyperthyroidism	TSH, triiodothyronine (T3), thyroxine (T4)

Management

Acute: start NS IV 3–4 L, Ca-losing diuretic (Lasix), cardiac monitoring, bisphosphonate, calcitonin.

Longer term: counsel the patient about the possible need for a parathyroidectomy.

Case 22: Claudication

A patient with a history of varicose veins has had claudication and calf pain for the past 6 months. Please perform a physical exam and interpret the patient's ECG. Give a differential diagnosis with risk factors, and recommend relevant investigations.

Time: 10 minutes

Physical exam

Be aware of the signs of critical ischemia.

Focus on the **5Ps**: **p**ain, **p**aresthesia, **p**allor, **p**aralysis, **p**ulselessness.

CATEGORY TO ASSESS	DETAILS
Vitals	BP (both arms, supine and upright)
	Pulse (carotid, brachial, radial, femoral, pedal): rate, rhythm, contour, amplitude, ankle brachial index (ABI)
HEENT	Xanthelasma
Heart	Murmur, signs of failure, increased jugular venous pressure
Extremities	Inspect: ulcer, skin color (pale, cyanotic), skin texture (atrophy), nail change/deformity, hair loss, muscle atrophy, edema, varicose veins
	Palpate (warmth/temperature, pulse quality): tender superficial veins, pitting edema, dependent rubor, pallor on elevation

Auscultate: carotid artery, renal arteries, abdominal aortic artery, iliac arteries, femoral arteries.

ECG interpretation

Look for left ventricular hypertrophy (LVH), old MI, and arrhythmia.

Differential diagnosis

POSSIBLE ETIOLOGY	SIGNS/SYMPTOMS
Arterial insufficiency	Calf discomfort on exertion, relieved by rest, reproducible pattern
	Signs of chronic ischemia distal to obstruction
Venous insufficiency	Standing: dilated, elongated superficial veins
	Supine: discoloration of shins (hemosiderin deposits), pitting edema, painless ulcers at the medial malleolus
	Trendelenburg test: valvular incompetence
Spinal stenosis/disc disease	Back pain, tenderness lateral to lumbosacral spine
	Lower extremities: restricted ROM, compromised sensory/motor/reflex responses, pain with straight-leg raise

Other differential diagnoses include cellulitis, deep vein thrombosis, phlegmasia alba dolens, and phlegmasia cerulea dolens.

RISK FACTORS FOR VASCULAR DISEASE

Risk factors include: smoking, HTN, coronary artery disease (CAD), DM, and hypercholesterol/lipidemia.

Investigations

Recommend, as appropriate: ABI, Doppler US, arteriogram, venogram, treadmill testing, lumbosacral spine X-ray, CT, MRI, and a workup for risk factors.

Case 23: Obesity

A 35-year-old man, who has been previously healthy other than obesity, is interested in losing weight. Please discuss management strategies with him.

Time: 5 minutes

History

Before you can offer a relevant management strategy, you need to take a history to understand factors that may affect the patient's obesity and his motivations for losing weight.

HISTORY OF PRESENT ILLNESS

How long have you been overweight?

What is your current weight?

What are the highest and lowest weights you have had as an adult?

Why do you want to lose weight now?

Do you have concerns about your self-image or health?

Do any of the following apply to you?

- snoring
- fatigue
- voice changes
- skin or hair changes
- cold intolerance
- swelling of the legs (edema)
- joint pain

How many times do you eat a day (snacks and meals)?

What do you eat (fat, fruit, vegetables, bread)?

When do you eat (e.g., while watching TV, before bed, at breakfast time, to relax, or when stressed)?

What do you do for exercise? How long? How often?

PAST MEDICAL HISTORY

Have you ever been diagnosed with any of the following?

- high blood pressure
- diabetes
- joint disease

What medications do you take?

Have you tried any weight-loss programs? What happened (effects, reasons for stopping)?

Is anyone else in your family overweight?

Is your family supportive about your plan to lose weight?

Management

Provide information about obesity:

- It increases the risk of high blood pressure, heart disease, gallbladder disease, fatty liver, DM, cancers (breast, bowel, cervix), osteoarthritis, sleep apnea, spinal dysfunction.
- It affects psychosocial well-being.
- Underlying diseases can cause it.
- Genetic factors influence weight, which we can't alter. But we can modify diet and exercise.

Counsel the patient about weight goals, diet, changing behaviors, exercise, and monitoring (see breakdown that follows).

COUNSELING CATEGORY	DETAILS
Weight goals	There is a range of healthy weights, no ideal weight.
	Set realistic goals for target weight and rate of loss.
Diet	Fad diets have no long-term benefits.
	To lose 0.5 kg/wk (1 lb/wk), reduce calorie intake by 300–500 kcal (1 g fat = 9 kcal, 1 g carbs = 4 kcal, 1 g protein = 4 kcal).
	Eat a balanced diet (follow the Canada Food Guide or the advice of a dietician).
	Have low calorie food available at all times for snacks.
Modifying food behaviors	Keep a food-intake diary.
	Eat only in one place.
	Don't do anything else while you eat (e.g., read, watch TV).
	Eat more slowly and use a smaller plate.
	Plan meals and shop from a list.
	At parties, avoid the food table.
Exercise	Begin with walking.
	Exercise at a specific time each day.
	Exercise for 30 minutes, 4–5 times per week, at 60% maximum heart rate (maximum heart rate = 200 – patient's age).
Monitoring	Self monitor.
	A support group can help.
	A buddy can help.

Refer the patient to a dietitian.

Discuss bariatric surgery, as appropriate.

Offer support (e.g., regular check-ups, consultation as needed).

Advise the patient to begin his food-intake diary immediately, and come back in a week to discuss it with you.

Case 24: Fatigue

A 35-year-old patient is experiencing fatigue. Please take a history, provide a differential diagnosis, recommend investigations, and outline a management plan.

Time: 10 minutes

History

HISTORY OF PRESENT ILLNESS

When did you begin feeling fatigued?

Did the fatigue start suddenly or gradually?

Are you experiencing stress in your life (e.g., grief, trauma, change in relationship, work, financial trouble, recent illness)?

How would you characterize the fatigue?

- Is it constant?
- Does it occur at certain times of day, or on certain days?
- Is there pain?

Have you noticed any changes in your symptoms lately?

What makes the fatigue better? Worse? Does it change with rest or exercise?

How does the fatigue affect your usual activities?

Are you experiencing any of the following?

- sleep changes: early waking, insomnia, snoring, sleep apnea, reflux when lying down
- appetite or weight changes
- fevers, sweats, swollen lymph nodes
- mood change, thoughts of suicide
- bowel habit changes, urinary changes, heat/cold intolerance
- muscle weakness

Are you pregnant, or could you be?

PAST MEDICAL HISTORY

Have you been diagnosed with any of the following?

- psychological disorders (e.g., depression, anxiety, eating disorder)
- diabetes
- lung disease
- hypertension
- liver or kidney disease
- rheumatologic disorders

What is the pattern of your sexual activity? (Assess risk for HIV.)

What medications do you take?

What is your family situation (e.g., chaotic, supportive)?

Do you smoke, drink, or use recreational drugs?

How old are you?

What do you do for a living?

Differential diagnosis

CATEGORY	POSSIBLE ETIOLOGY
Psychogenic disorder	Depression, anxiety, somatization disorder, personality disorder, eating disorder
Pharmaceuticals	Hypnotics, antihypertensives, antidepressants, tranquilizers, street drugs
Endocrine disorder	Diabetes, hypothyroidism, pituitary insufficiency, Addison disease, renal/liver failure
Unknown etiology	Chronic fatigue syndrome
Anemia	Malignancy
Infection	Endocarditis, TB, HIV, mononucleosis
Connective tissue disease	Rheumatoid arthritis, SLE
Disturbed sleep	Sleep apnea, gastroesophageal reflux, allergic rhinitis
Muscle weakness	Myasthenia gravis
Pregnancy	
Cardiac/pulmonary failure	CHF, MI

Investigations

Recommend, as appropriate:

- CBC, electrolytes, ESR, glucose, TSH, urinalysis, CXR, ECG, beta-hCG
- serology: Epstein-Barr virus (EBV), CMV, HIV, HBsAg, VDRL

Management

Treat the cause.

If chronic fatigue syndrome: administer low dose antidepressants, NSAIDs.

If undetermined etiology: reassure; follow up; recommend exercise, behavior/group therapy; administer vitamins.

Case 25: Skin rashes, blisters

A 21-year-old woman presents with a skin rash. Please obtain a focused history and perform a physical exam.

Time: 10 minutes

History

HISTORY OF PRESENT ILLNESS

When did the rash develop?

Did it develop suddenly or gradually?

Where is it?

Is the rash itchy or painful?

Is there any discharge from it (e.g., blood, pus)?

Has the rash changed over time (extent, qualities)?

Have you had any topical or oral medications recently?

Did you have any symptoms before the rash developed (e.g., fever, sore throat, loss of appetite, vaginal discharge, joint pain, swelling)?

Do any of the following apply to you?

- recent travel
- insect bites
- exposure to toxins (environmental, domestic, industrial)

Have you had close contact with anyone who has a skin rash?

PAST MEDICAL HISTORY

Have you had this before?

Do you have a history of skin disease?

Do you have allergies?

What medications are you taking?

Has anyone in your family been diagnosed with a skin disease or other diseases?

What is the pattern of your sexual activity? (Assess risk for STD, HIV.)

Do you use recreational drugs? (Assess risk for HIV.)

How old are you?

What do you do for a living?

What do you do for recreation (e.g., sports, hobbies)?

Physical exam

Inspect the rash for:

- distribution and arrangement, symmetry
- lesion size, shape, location, configuration, uniformity, pedunculation
- elevation or depression, swelling

Palpate the rash for: moisture, temperature, turgor, texture, and blanching.

Inspect the skin for:

- thickness
- hygiene, odors, exudates

Examine the hair, mucus membranes, nails, thyroid, and lymph nodes.

Palpate the abdomen for hepatosplenomegaly.

Case 26: Joint pain

A patient is experiencing joint pain. Please take a history, do a physical exam, provide a differential diagnosis, and recommend relevant investigations.

Time: 10 minutes

History

The history should focus on distinguishing the following possible conditions:

- articular versus nonarticular
- inflammatory versus degenerative arthritis
- focal versus global; local versus systemic (e.g., septic arthritis)

HISTORY OF PRESENT ILLNESS

When did the joint pain start?

Where is the pain?

- Where is it most intense?
- Is it on one side of your body or both sides?
- Does it radiate to other parts of your body?

What is the pain like (e.g., sharp, aching)?

When do you have pain (e.g., time of day, certain days)?

Does anything make the pain better?

What were you doing when the pain started?

Do you have any of the following symptoms? (See breakdown that follows.)

SYMPTOM/FACTOR	POSSIBLE ETIOLOGY
Morning stiffness lasting more than 30 minutes	Inflammatory
Tenderness, swelling, redness, warmth	
Improvement with exercise	
Worse later in day	Mechanical/degenerative
Better with rest	
Locking, giving way, instability	
Constant pain, night pain	Neoplastic/infectious
Fever, sweats	
Loss of appetite, weight loss, fatigue	

Do you have a rash?

Do you have any insect bites?

PAST MEDICAL HISTORY

Have you had this pain before?

- If yes, how has it behaved over time (e.g., intermittent over the years, gradually worsening over time, or waxing/waning with slow progression over time)?

How is the pain affecting your daily activities (e.g., getting up, using the bathroom, combing your hair)?

Do you have a history of problems with any of the following?

- skin
- kidneys/urinary system (especially if pain radiates to the back)
- eyes
- lungs
- stomach/digestive system
- heart (especially if pain radiates from the chest to the shoulder, neck, or arm)

Have you ever been diagnosed with any of the following cancers: (mnemonic: **PT B**arnum **L**oves **K**ids) **p**rostate, **t**hyroid, **b**reast, **l**ung, **k**idney?

What medications do you take?

Has anyone in your family been diagnosed with a joint or autoimmune disease?

What is the pattern of your sexual activity? (Assess risk for STDs.)

How old are you?

What do you do for a living?

Physical exam

CATEGORY TO ASSESS	DETAILS
Vitals	Note if fever
Joints	Examine above and below affected joint
	Inspect:
	• shape, alignment, position at rest, discoloration
	• (mnemonic: **SEADS**) **s**welling, **e**rythema, muscle **a**trophy, **d**eformity, **s**kin changes
	Palpate: temperature, tenderness, effusion, crepitus, laxity/instability; soft tissue, bursa
	Test ROM: if passive ROM is greater than active ROM, suggests soft tissue inflammation or muscle weakness
Neurovascular system	Check: power, pulses, reflexes, sensation, fasciculations

(*Continued*)

CATEGORY TO ASSESS	DETAILS
Special tests	Lachlan test, McMurray test
Gait/posture	Observe walking: heel to toe, on heels, on toes Note if: Trendelenburg gait (hip disorders), antalgic gait, high stepping, circumduction

Differential diagnosis

See Table 12.

Table 12. DIFFERENTIAL DIAGNOSIS OF JOINT PAIN

TYPE	POSSIBLE ETIOLOGY
Inflammatory articular	Rheumatoid arthritis, SLE, scleroderma, psoriatic, reactive, ankylosing spondylitis, gout, gonococcal, Lyme disease, bacterial endocarditis
Noninflammatory articular	Osteoarthritis, hypertrophic pulmonary osteoarthropathy, myxedema, amyloidosis
Inflammatory periarticular	Polymyalgia rheumatica, dermatomyositis, eosinophilia-myalgia syndrome
Noninflammatory periarticular	Fibromyalgia, reflex sympathetic dystrophy

TIPS FOR DIFFERENTIATION

CONDITION	CLINICAL PRESENTATION
Articular versus nonarticular	Location, aggravating/releasing factors, functional loss
Inflammatory versus noninflammatory	Redness, warmth, swelling, tenderness X-ray: • inflammatory shows diffuse erosion • noninflammatory shows cartilage loss, decreased joint space, bony overgrowth, erosions
Rheumatoid arthritis	< 40-year-old women (more so than men), morning stiffness, Raynaud syndrome, fever
Ankylosing spondylitis	< 40-year-old men (more so than women)
Sjogren	Dry mouth and eyes
Gout	Men, postmenopausal women
Reactive	Men, conjunctivitis, urethritis
SLE	Premenopausal women, Raynaud syndrome
Fibromyalgia	Chronic fatigue, sleep disorder, focal tender points

Associated symptoms can also help with differentiation:

- rash: SLE, gonococcus, Lyme disease, vasculitis, psoriatic
- fever: septic joint, allergy, rheumatoid arthritis, SLE, bacterial endocarditis
- diarrhea: inflammatory bowel disease

Investigations

INVESTIGATION CATEGORY	DETAILS
General chemistry	CBC, electrolytes, BUN, Cr, urate
Acute phase reactants	ESR, C3, C4, fibrinogen, CRP, albumin
Serology	RF, ANA, antigen-antibody (Ag-Ab) complexes
Synovial fluid	Gross appearance (volume, color, clarity, viscosity), cell count and differential, crystals, culture, and sensitivity
Cultures	Urinalysis, GU cultures
X-ray	X-ray of affected joints

Case 27: Hair loss

A 40-year-old man is experiencing hair loss. Please take a history.

Time: 5 minutes

History

HISTORY OF PRESENT ILLNESS

When did the hair loss begin?

Was it sudden or gradual?

Does it occur only on the scalp or is body hair involved as well?

Is the baldness localized or generalized? Symmetric or asymmetric?

Have you experienced any of the following recently?

- high fever
- weight loss
- severe illness
- emotional stress
- female patients: pregnancy

PAST MEDICAL HISTORY

Have you ever been diagnosed with a thyroid disorder?

What medications are you taking?

Does anyone in your family have baldness or hair loss? Women or men?

Case 28: Weight loss

An 80-year-old man presents with recent weight loss. Please take a history, do a physical exam, and recommend investigations.

Time: 10 minutes

History

HISTORY OF PRESENT ILLNESS

How much weight have you lost? Over how long (weeks, months, years)?

Is the weight loss intentional?

Do you enjoy your meals? How is your appetite?

What is your usual diet (breakfast, lunch, supper)?

Does eating cause pain or discomfort?

Do any of the following apply to you?

- nausea, vomiting, abdominal pain
- other pain
- changes in bowel habits or stool (consistency, color)
- fever, night sweats, tremor, weather intolerance
- increased urine volume, excessive thirst
- cough
- mass or lump
- changes in your fingernails

Are you experiencing stress in your life?

PAST MEDICAL HISTORY

Have you been diagnosed with any illnesses?

Have you recently started or stopped any medications?

What conditions or illnesses run in your family?

Are you or have you been an alcoholic?

Do you have a history of smoking?

Do you have a history of using recreational drugs?

Physical exam

CATEGORY	DETAILS
General	Evidence of weight loss, cachexia, wasting, hair loss, calloused knuckles, nail changes
HEENT	Thyroid, lymphadenopathy (especially supraclavicular), oropharynx, loss of tooth enamel
Respiratory system	Evidence of chronic obstructive pulmonary disease (COPD), other lung disease
Cardiovascular system	Heart rate, BP, air entry, wheezes
Breasts, axilla	Masses, lymphadenopathy
Abdomen	Ascites, hepatosplenomegaly, inguinal lymphadenopathy

Investigations

Recommend:

- general chemistry: CBC, liver function tests
- CXR if indicated
- CT chest/abdomen if indicated

Case 29: Sore throat

A 60-year-old woman visits your office because she has a sore throat. Please obtain a focused history.

Time: 5 minutes

History

HISTORY OF PRESENT ILLNESS

How long have you had a sore throat?

Did it develop suddenly or slowly?

Does anything make the pain worse or better?

What is the pain like (e.g., localized or diffuse, constant or changing in severity)?

Do you have any of the following symptoms?

- lung symptoms (e.g., cough, sputum)
- ear, nose and throat symptoms (e.g., sinus pain, postnasal drip, ear pain)
- hoarseness, difficulty swallowing
- acid reflux, regurgitation into the mouth (water brash)

What medications do you take?

Do you use intraoral steroids?

Are you sexually active? Do you have unprotected oral sex?

Do you drink alcohol? If so, how much and how often?

Do you have a history of smoking?

Case 30: Ankle edema

A patient presents with bilateral ankle edema. Please take a history, do a physical exam, provide a differential diagnosis, recommend investigations, and outline an initial management strategy.

Time: 10 minutes

History

HISTORY OF PRESENT ILLNESS

How long have you had the swelling?

Did it develop suddenly or gradually?

Does the swelling change during the day (e.g., better in the morning or in the afternoon)?

Does anything alleviate the swelling (e.g., rest, ice)?

Does anything make the swelling worse (e.g., certain activities)?

What activity were you doing just before the swelling began?

Do any of the following factors or conditions apply to you?

- trauma to the legs associated with redness, pain, fever
- recent surgery
- calf pain that consistently develops with exertion and is relieved by rest (vascular claudication symptoms)
- leg problems: pain, tingling/burning/numbness, weakness, loss of function (neurological claudication)
- joint problems
- cold intolerance (hypothyroidism)
- shortness of breath, chest pain (pulmonary embolism, CHF)
- jaundice, indigestion, bleeding problems (liver disease)
- blood in the urine (hematuria), facial/eyelid swelling, recent sore throat (kidney)
- diarrhea, foul-smelling stools (GI)

Are you pregnant or have you been recently pregnant?

PAST MEDICAL HISTORY

Have you had previous episodes of swelling in your ankles?

- How long did the swelling last?
- How did it resolve?

Have you been diagnosed with any of the following?

- varicose veins, phlebitis, deep vein thrombosis
- myocardial infarction
- congestive heart failure
- pulmonary embolism, thrombophilia
- cancer
- kidney disease
- liver disease
- thyroid disease
- protein in the urine (proteinuria)
- inability to absorb nutrients from your food (malabsorption)

What medications do you take?

Are you taking any new medications?

Do you take birth control pills?

Do you have any allergies?

Have you been hospitalized recently?

What is your diet like? (Assess the quality of the patient's nutrition.)

Are you an alcoholic?

Physical exam

CATEGORY	DETAILS
Inspection	General appearance, cachexia
	Face: jaundice, eyelid swelling
	Skin: color, cyanosis, spider nevi, bruising
	Neck: thyroid mass, jugular venous pressure
	Chest: symmetry, shape, gynecomastia
	Abdomen: shape, ascites, scars, caput medusa
	GU: scrotal swelling
	Extremities: microcirculation, edema (degree and extent on both sides), lymph nodes, varicose veins, deep vein insufficiency

(Continued)

CATEGORY	DETAILS
Palpation	Thyroid, lymph nodes, pain, mass, hepatic-jugular reflux
Percussion	Heart, lungs, liver, costovertebral angle (CVA) tenderness, ascites, pleural effusion
Auscultation	Heart (S3), lungs, thyroid for bruits, renal artery bruits, bowel sounds

Differential diagnosis

See Table 13.

Table 13. DIFFERENTIAL DIAGNOSIS OF BILATERAL ANKLE EDEMA

TYPE	POSSIBLE ETIOLOGY
Oncotic pressure	Malnutrition, liver failure, nephrotic syndrome, protein-losing enteropathy, cancer
Hydrostatic pressure	CHF, renal failure, venous insufficiency, pregnancy, menstruation
Capillary permeability	Systemic vasculitis, idiopathic edema, allergy
Lymphatic obstruction	Retroperitoneal, generalized
Endocrine disorder	Myxedema, Grave disease
Iatrogenic disorder	MAOI, antihypertensives, corticosteroids, estrogen, progesterone, NSAIDs
Trauma	Damage to lymphatics or venous drainage

Investigations

ETIOLOGY	INVESTIGATIONS
Heart disease	CXR, ECG, CBC, electrolytes, lipid profile
Thyroid disease	TSH
Kidney disease	Cr, urinalysis
Liver disease	Liver function tests, serum albumin

Management

Treat the underlying cause.

Counsel the patient to:

- Restrict salt intake.
- Avoid prolonged standing or sitting, and to elevate legs.
- Use support stockings.
- Avoid salt-retaining drugs (e.g., certain diuretics).

Depending on etiology, prescribe:

- diuretics
- heparin for deep vein thrombosis
- prednisone 1 mg/kg × 4–8 wk for minimal change disease of kidney

Case 31: AIDS

A patient with HIV needs treatment for recently diagnosed *Pneumocystis jiroveci*. Please perform a physical exam and outline a management strategy.

Time: 5 minutes

Physical exam

The physical exam needs to focus on signs of infection or malignancy that indicate the development of AIDS.

CATEGORY TO ASSESS	FINDINGS TO NOTE IF PRESENT
Vitals	Fever, hypotension
General appearance	Septic shock, malnutrition, dehydration, cyanosis (central/peripheral)
Skin and mucus membranes	Hydration: dry mucous membranes, decreased turgor Rashes: • Kaposi sarcoma: skin and oral mucosa • herpes simplex/herpes zoster: nasolabial, genital, chest wall • warts: molluscum contagiosum, human papilloma virus (HPV), hairy cell leukemia • morbilliform eruption • seborrheic dermatitis • eosinophilic pustular folliculitis • bacterial/fungal infections: erythema, swelling, pain, warmth
HEENT	Eyes: CMV retinitis
	Oral cavity: hairy leukoplakia, thrush, mucosal petechiae, stomatitis, gingivitis, Kaposi sarcoma, angular cheilitis
	Nasal discharge: sinus infection
Lymph nodes	Persistent generalized lymphadenopathy

(Continued)

CATEGORY TO ASSESS	FINDINGS TO NOTE IF PRESENT
Heart	Murmurs and rubs: pericarditis, myocarditis, endocarditis
Jugular venous pressure	Cor pulmonale, bounding pulse
Lungs	Inspection: respiratory distress, breathing pattern, respiratory depth and rhythm, chest wall deformity/inequality
	Percussion: dullness, consolidation, pleural effusion/ inflammation, hyperresonance
	Palpation: crepitus, fremitus, excursion
	Auscultation: vocal resonance, whisper pectoriloquy, adventitious sound
Extremities	Arthritis, vasculitis, sensory/motor dysfunction
	Clubbing
	Edema: CHF
Neurological	Meningitis/encephalitis: meningeal irritation, focal deficits
	Mental status: dementia
	Peripheral neuropathy/myopathy
Abdomen	Liver, spleen: masses, tenderness
Genitourinary system	Ulcerations, swelling, discharge, papillomatous
	DRE, Pap test

Management

For *Pneumocystis jiroveci*, administer:

- oxygen to maintain oxygen saturation above 90%
- trimetoprima/sulfamethoxazole

Treat HIV with appropriate combinations of antiretroviral drugs.

Case 32: Repeated epistaxis and skin bruises

A 30-year-old woman has had repeated epistaxis and skin bruises. Please take a history, perform a physical exam, provide a differential diagnosis, and recommend investigations.

Time: 10 minutes

History

HISTORY OF PRESENT ILLNESS

How often do you get nosebleeds?

Are the nosebleeds spontaneous or traumatic?

Are you having difficulty breathing or a sensation of nasal obstruction?

How quickly does the bleeding stop? What needs to be done to stop the bleeding?

When did you notice bruising on your skin?

Where was the bruising?

How often do you have bruising?

How does the bruising occur (spontaneously or because of trauma)?

How does it resolve? How long does it take?

If you have bleeding with an injury, what is the bleeding like?

Do any of the following factors or conditions apply to you?

- current upper respiratory tract infection
- exposure to dry heat
- nose picking
- forceful nose blowing
- current liver, kidney, or bone marrow disease

Are you experiencing any of the following?

- pain
- fever
- weight loss
- swollen lymph nodes
- night sweats
- heavy menstrual bleeding
- blood in your stools

PAST MEDICAL HISTORY

What medications do you take?

Has anyone in your family been diagnosed with a bleeding disorder?

What illnesses run in your family?

How old are you?

What do you do for a living?

Physical exam

CATEGORY TO ASSESS	DETAILS
Vitals	BP, jugular venous pressure (R/O serious hemorrhage or volume depletion)
General condition	Cushingoid or marfanoid appearance
Systemic disease	Septicemia, fever, toxic anemia, lymphadenopathy, splenomegaly, hematoma and hemarthroses in joints and muscles
Skin and mucus membranes	Petechiae < 3 cm, purpura < 1 cm, ecchymosis > 3 cm (size, number, location)
	Spider nevi, telangiectasia
	Vascular insufficiency
GI system	Bleeding (DRE)

Differential diagnosis

See Table 14.

Table 14. DIFFERENTIAL DIAGNOSIS OF BLEEDING DISORDERS

TYPE	POSSIBLE ETIOLOGY
Qualitative	Von Willebrand disease, NSAID use
Quantitative	Increased destruction: ITP, TTP, vasculitis, drug, immune/nonimmune, splenic sequestration, hypersplenism
	Decreased production: marrow disease, aplastic anemia, fibrosis, lymphoma/leukemia, myelodysplastic syndrome, multiple myeloma
Coagulation factor	Extrinsic: vitamin K deficiency, anticoagulant use
	Intrinsic: hemophilia A, B
Vascular factor	Scurvy, Cushing syndrome, drug-induced platelet dysfunction, hereditary platelet disorder, connective tissue disease
Systemic	Renal failure, liver failure, disseminated intravascular coagulation, HIV

Investigations

INVESTIGATION CATEGORY	DETAILS
Platelet count	CBC, peripheral smear, platelet count
Factor deficiency, anticoagulant use	PT, PTT
Platelet quality	Aggregation test, ristocetin-induced agglutination
Thrombocytopenia etiology	Bone marrow aspirate/biopsy, platelet bound IgG autoantibody, HIV serology, urine and serum electrophoresis
Coagulation factor production	LFTs, renal function tests (RFTs), FDP, ESR

Case 33: Hand weakness

A patient presents with unilateral right hand weakness. Please take a history, provide a differential diagnosis, and recommend investigations.

Time: 5 minutes

History

The history should focus on differentiating systemic disease from localized disease.

HISTORY OF PRESENT ILLNESS

When did the hand weakness start?

Did it develop suddenly or gradually?

Does it happen at particular times of day (e.g., in the morning, after activity)?

How has it changed over time (e.g., stayed the same, fluctuated, become worse)?

Have you injured your arm recently (trauma)?

Are areas of your body affected besides your hand?

Are both hands weak, or just one?

Is the weakness closer to the center of your body, or closer to the tips of your extremities (proximal or distal)?

Do you have any of the following symptoms in your hand or arm?

- pain
- numbness
- stiffness
- floppiness

Do you have joint pain in your arm?

Which hand is your dominant hand?

Are you having problems with any of the following?

- arms generally
- facial expression
- vision
- gait

Have you had any of the following recently?

- injuries
- infections
- fever or weight loss

PAST MEDICAL HISTORY

Have you been diagnosed with any illnesses?

What medications do you take?

Have you ever been hospitalized for any conditions?

Does your family have a history of any of the following conditions?

- muscle disease
- high blood pressure
- diabetes
- heart disease
- neurological disorders
- psychological disorders
- seizures
- stroke

Differential diagnosis

See Table 15.

Table 15. DIFFERENTIAL DIAGNOSIS OF UNILATERAL HAND WEAKNESS

CATEGORY	POSSIBLE ETIOLOGY
Neurologic	Central: stroke
	Peripheral: disc, C-spine, carpal tunnel
Vascular	Claudication, thoracic outlet syndrome
Muscular	Trauma, myopathy
Endocrine	Myasthenia gravis, hypothyroidism, Cushing syndrome

(Continued)

Table 15. (*Continued*)

CATEGORY	POSSIBLE ETIOLOGY
Metabolic	Hyponatremia, hypocalcemia
Space-occupying lesion	Tumor
Connective tissue disease	Polymyositis, dermatomyositis

Investigations

INVESTIGATION CATEGORY	DETAILS
Blood	CBC, electrolytes, PTT/INR, VDRL, glucose, lipids
Imaging studies	C-spine, arm, CT, MRI
Vessels	Doppler, angiography (carotids)
Cardiac	ECG, echocardiogram
Neuropathy/myopathy	Creatine kinase, nerve conduction studies, electromyography, muscle biopsy

Obstetrics and gynecology

Case 34: Amenorrhea

A 30-year-old woman presents with amenorrhea. Please obtain a focused history and recommend investigations.

Time: 5 minutes

History

The history needs to first establish whether the condition is primary or secondary amenorrhea, and then move to appropriate focused questions.

HISTORY OF PRESENT ILLNESS

Have you ever had periods?

FOCUSED QUESTIONS: PRIMARY AMENORRHEA

Have you had the following?

- breast development
- pubic/axillary hair development
- growth spurt

What is your growth history, including weight gain?

Have you suffered stressful life events or abuse?

Is there a history in your family of delayed puberty, delayed menarche, or infertility?

FOCUSED QUESTIONS: SECONDARY AMENORRHEA

How many periods have you missed? When was your last menstrual period?

Were your periods regular before? If not, how irregular were they?

Is this the first time your period has stopped?

Do you think you might be pregnant? Do you have nausea or vomiting? Breast tenderness? Urinary frequency?

Do you think you might be menopausal? How old are you? Do you have hot flashes or vaginal dryness?

Do you have any of the following symptoms?

- vision changes
- changes in your sense of smell
- headache
- changes in libido
- weight gain
- cold intolerance
- increased fatigue
- increased or excessive hair growth
- acne
- easy bruising
- muscle weakness
- high blood pressure
- voice changes
- obesity centered on the trunk/abdomen (truncal/central obesity)

How much exercise do you do? Have you lost weight?

PAST MEDICAL HISTORY
(PRIMARY AND SECONDARY AMENORRHEA)

Are you taking any medications? Are you taking birth control pills or hormone replacement therapy?

Have you had radiation therapy?

Have you had any gynecological procedures (e.g., loop electrosurgical excision procedure, hysterectomy)?

Have you had any STDs?

Have you ever been pregnant? If so, how many times?

Have you miscarried and, if so, at what stage of pregnancy?

Have you had problems getting pregnant? Have you used any conception aids?

How many children do you have?

Do you know the menstrual history of your female relatives (mother, sister)?

What is the pattern of your sexual activity?

Have you experienced any stress, depression, bereavement, or major life
events?

Investigations

FOR SECONDARY AMENORRHEA

The most important cause of secondary amenorrhea is pregnancy, so every
workup should start with a urine or serum beta-hCG.

Following a negative pregnancy test, the next diagnostic maneuver is a
progesterone challenge (Provera 10 mg/dL orally × 5–10 d). If a withdrawal
bleed results, this is diagnostic of hypothalamic amenorrhea.

If no withdrawal bleed results, look for other causes by measuring:

- LH and FSH (low in pituitary defect, FSH high in ovarian defects)
- TSH (low in hypothyroidism)
- dehydroepiandrosterone (DHEA), testosterone (high in polycystic
  ovarian syndrome)
- CT or MRI to rule out pituitary adenoma or empty sella syndrome
- pelvic US to look for outflow obstruction

Investigations should also include a focused physical exam: appearance
(cachexia, obese, cushingoid, hirsute, secondary sexual characteristics), visual
fields, breast exam, pelvic exam.

FOR PRIMARY AMENORRHEA

Investigations for primary amenorrhea are similar to those for secondary
amenorrhea but also include:

- a karyotype to rule out Turner syndrome
- serum testosterone to rule out complete androgen resistance (testicular
  feminization)

Case 35: Menorrhagia

A 41-year-old woman has had heavy vaginal bleeding for the past 3 periods. Please take a history, provide a differential diagnosis, recommend investigations, and outline a management plan.

Time: 5 minutes

History

HISTORY OF PRESENT ILLNESS

Before this problem began, what was your usual pattern of menstrual bleeding (length, duration, volume)?

When did it start to change? Did it change gradually or suddenly? Do you have any suspected cause?

What is your current pattern of menstrual bleeding (length, duration, volume)? Is the heavy bleeding getting better or worse?

Do you have bleeding at other times (e.g., between periods, after intercourse)?

Do you have any of the following symptoms?

- dizziness, black outs, palpitations (anemia)
- fever, vaginal discharge, pain with urination, pain with intercourse, abdominal pain (infection)
- weight loss (malignancy)
- unusual growth of body hair (hirsutism)
- nipple discharge (galactorrhea)
- slow movement, heat/cold intolerance, constipation (hypothyroidism)
- pelvic pain (infection, torsion, degenerated fibroid, atrophic vaginitis)

Is it possible that you are pregnant?

Do you experience any changes when you ovulate (e.g., mood changes)?

Have you been experiencing bruising or excessive bleeding at other sites?

PAST MEDICAL HISTORY

Have you seen a doctor for this problem before?

Do you use contraceptives (IUD, oral contraceptive)?

Have you used clomifene?

What medications do you take (e.g., steroids, antidepressants, antipsychotics, anticoagulants)?

Have you ever been diagnosed with any of the following?

- kidney or liver disease
- coagulation disorder
- diabetes
- obesity
- hypothyroidism
- pelvic disorders

What is the pattern of your sexual activity? (Assess for STD risk.)

How old are you?

Differential diagnosis

See Table 16.

Table 16. DIFFERENTIAL DIAGNOSIS OF MENORRHAGIA

CATEGORY	POSSIBLE ETIOLOGY
Complications of pregnancy	Infection, retained products of conception
Anovulation	Menopause, oligomenorrhea, pregnancy
Neoplasia	Benign: polyps, leiomyomata, endometrial hyperplasia, endometriosis
	Malignant: endometrial cancer, cervical cancer, ovarian cancer
Infection	Cervicitis, endometritis, STDs
Trauma	Iatrogenic procedures, radiation, rape, foreign body
Nongynecological condition	Coagulopathy, liver disease, SLE
Endocrine disorder	Hypothyroidism, prolactinemia, Cushing syndrome, polycystic ovary syndrome (PCOS), adrenal dysfunction, adrenal tumor

Investigations

Recommend:

- CBC, PTT, INR, LH, FSH, TSH, pregnancy test, progesterone
- Pap smear, STD swabs of cervix
- transvaginal US

In perimenopausal patients, recommend an endometrial biopsy and vaginal US for endometrial thickness.

In premenopausal patients, evaluate anovulation (see Case 34).

Management

Treat according to etiology.

For diagnosed anovulatory cycles without hypothalamic causes, prescribe birth control pills.

For anemia, prescribe birth control pills and progesterone support as appropriate.

If menorrhagia persists, the patient may need a hysteroscopy, D&C, endometrial US, and endometrial biopsy.

For symptomatic anemia or if hemoglobin is unstable, recommend a transfusion and a D&C.

Case 36: Vaginal bleeding

A 40-year-old woman presents with vaginal bleeding. Please obtain a history and provide a differential diagnosis.

Time: 5 minutes

History

HISTORY OF PRESENT ILLNESS

When did the vaginal bleeding begin?

Did it develop suddenly or gradually?

Has it changed over time?

How many pads or tampons do you need when the bleeding is happening?

Does anything make the bleeding worse or better?

Is there an odor with the blood? Are there clots or tissue?

Do you have abdominal cramps or pain?

Do you have a fever?

Are you pregnant or could you be? (Ask about unprotected sex, breast engorgement, fatigue, urinary frequency, nausea and vomiting.)

If not pregnant, are you experiencing any of the following symptoms?

- postcoital bleeding, fever, weight loss (malignancy)
- dizziness, shortness of breath, blackouts (anemia)
- belly pain, fever, vaginal discharge, urinary frequency, pain with intercourse (STD)

If pregnant:

- Have you been treated for vaginal bleeding before?
- Have you had an ultrasound? (Ask about placental position, growth.)
- Have you ever been diagnosed with anemia?

PAST MEDICAL HISTORY

Do any of the following conditions or factors apply to you?

- unusual growth of body hair (e.g., face, chest)
- infertility
- special diet
- obesity

Do you bleed easily (bleeding diathesis)?

Are you on medications inhibiting normal clotting (e.g., blood thinner)?

What is your normal menstrual period like (regularity, amount, intermenstrual bleeding)?

When was your last menstrual period?

Have you had previous pregnancies (including full-term pregnancies, miscarriages, therapeutic abortions)?

Have you ever been diagnosed with an STD?

Do you use contraception (IUD, oral contraceptive)?

Have you had a Pap smear? When? What were the results?

Do you drink, smoke, or use recreational drugs?

Are you experiencing stress in your life?

Differential diagnosis

Possible etiologies of vaginal bleeding include:

- perimenopausal bleeding
- neoplasia (cervix, vagina, endometrium)
- polyps (cervix, endometrium)
- trauma
- infection
- coagulopathy
- pregnancy (threatened abortion, ectopic, molar, fetal loss)

Case 37: Vaginal bleeding during pregnancy

A woman who is 7 weeks pregnant presents with vaginal bleeding and lower abdominal pain. Please obtain a focused history, provide a differential diagnosis with treatment options, and outline appropriate investigations.

Time: 5 minutes

History

HISTORY OF PRESENT ILLNESS

When did the bleeding begin?

Did it develop suddenly or gradually?

Has it changed over time?

How many pads or tampons do you need when the bleeding is happening?

Does anything make the bleeding worse or better?

Is there an odor with the blood? Are there clots or tissue?

Do you have abdominal cramps or pain?

Do you have a fever?

Have you been treated for vaginal bleeding before?

Have you had an ultrasound? (Ask about placental position, growth.)

PAST MEDICAL HISTORY

Have you had any of the following?

- uterine surgery or structural abnormality
- anemia
- STD
- coagulation abnormalities
- autoimmune disease

Do you bleed easily (bleeding diathesis)?

What medications are you taking?

Have you had previous pregnancies? How many full-term pregnancies, miscarriages, and therapeutic abortions?

Have you had a Pap smear? When? What were the results?

Do you have a family history of coagulation or autoimmune disease?

Do you drink, smoke, or use recreational drugs?

Differential diagnosis

See Table 17.

Table 17. DIFFERENTIAL DIAGNOSIS AND TREATMENT OF VAGINAL BLEEDING DURING PREGNANCY

ETIOLOGY	MANAGEMENT
Threatened abortion	US for viability of fetus
Incomplete or inevitable abortion	D&C with or without oxytocin
Complete abortion	No treatment
Septic abortion	D&C, antibiotic, oxygen
Ectopic pregnancy	Methotrexate, surgery
Molar pregnancy	Surgery, chemotherapy
Cervical polyp, genital cancer	Surgery
Physiological bleeding (placental development)	Emotional support, observation

Possible causes of repeated spontaneous abortions include:

- uterine abnormalities:
  - leiomyoma
  - adhesions
  - congenital malformation
- anticardiolipin antibody syndrome
- chromosomal imbalance
- exogenous substances:
  - IUD
  - methotrexate
  - NSAIDs
  - retinoids
  - toxins: organic solvents, heavy metals, alcohol, ethylene glycol

Investigations

Rule out bleeding vaginal or cervical lesions: speculum examination.

Rule out molar and ectopic pregnancy in all patients with early pregnancy bleeding: US, beta-hCG.

In the case of recurrent spontaneous abortions:

- Look for chromosomal abnormalities (Turner syndrome, autosomal or X-linked dominant or recessive diseases) through genetic analysis (karyotype).
- Check for anticardiolipin antibodies.

Case 38: Vaginal discharge

A woman presents with bloody vaginal discharge. Please obtain a history, give a differential diagnosis, and recommend investigations.

Time: 5 minutes

History

The odor, color, and timing of the discharge are important.

HISTORY OF PRESENT ILLNESS

How long has the discharge been present?

Do you need a pad or liner to manage it? How many per day?

What is the discharge like (color, consistency, odor)?

- Is it sticky or cheesy?
- Is it blood-stained?

When does the discharge happen (e.g., after intercourse, midcycle)?

Do you have any of the following symptoms?

- abdominal pain or fever
- itching or burning of the vulvar area
- urinary changes (pain, hesitancy, urgency, need to urinate at night)
- pain with intercourse
- skin rashes

Do you have unprotected sex?

Do you have a new sexual partner?

Does your partner have a discharge?

Have you experienced weight loss, coughing, or bone pain in your lower back?

PAST MEDICAL HISTORY

Have you had any of the following?

- STD
- vaginal infection

Do you have diabetes?

Do you have allergies?

What is your normal menstrual period like (regularity, amount, intermenstrual bleeding)?

When was your last menstrual period?

Have you had previous pregnancies (including full-term pregnancies, miscarriages, therapeutic abortions)?

Do you use contraception (IUD, oral contraceptive)?

Have you had a Pap smear? When? What were the results?

What is your vaginal hygiene routine (e.g., bubble bath, genital deodorants, soaps, use of wipes, douching, clothing habits)?

Differential diagnosis

See Table 18.

Table 18. DIFFERENTIAL DIAGNOSIS OF VAGINAL DISCHARGE

CATEGORY	POSSIBLE ETIOLOGY
Infection	STD: gonorrhea, herpes, chlamydia, trichomoniasis, pelvic inflammatory disease
	Non-STD: *Candida*, bacterial vaginosis (*Gardnerella*)
Physiologic hormonal change	Leucorrhea, atrophic vaginitis
Other	Chemical allergy, foreign body, IUD, cancer, polyp, cervicitis

Management

Counsel the patient to avoid nylon underwear, pantyhose, wet bathing suits, tight jeans, abrasive soaps.

Explain that barrier contraception results in safer sex.

If the patient has an STD, provide appropriate treatment to the patient and treat the patient's partner (see breakdown that follows). Counsel the patient to avoid sex during treatment.

STD	TREATMENT
Trichomonas vaginalis	Metronidazole 2 g po once
Gardnerella vaginalis	If symptomatic or pregnant: metronidazole 500 mg po bid × 7 days
Chlamydia trachomatis	Doxycycline 100 mg bid × 7 days or azithromycin 1 g po once
Neisseria gonorrhea	Ciprofloxacin 500 mg po once
Candida	Fluconazole cream or oral antifungal medication

If the patient has a coinfection with HIV, a longer treatment course is required. Refer the patient to an infectious disease specialist.

Report STDs to your public health authority.

Investigations

Recommend:

- analysis of vaginal secretions: C&S, saline wet mount, KOH wet mount, pH
- smear microscopy, Gram stain

Case 39: Prenatal testing for aneuploidy counseling

A 37-year-old woman is 9 weeks pregnant and concerned about trisomy 21. Please take a history and discuss a management plan with her.

Time: 5 minutes

History

The history needs to assess the risk for trisomy 21, and also for other gestational and genetic abnormalities.

HISTORY OF PRESENT ILLNESS

What is your age?

Are you certain you are pregnant? (Ask about fatigue, nausea and vomiting, backache, groin pain, constipation, pregnancy test.)

When was your last menstrual period (LMP)? (Determine expected delivery date (EDD): EDD = LMP + 7 days – 3 months.)

Is this your first pregnancy?

Is this a planned pregnancy?

PAST MEDICAL HISTORY

Have you been diagnosed with any of the following?

- high blood pressure
- type 2 diabetes
- heart disease
- liver disease
- kidney disease
- epilepsy
- HIV
- viral hepatitis

What is your ethnicity?

Does your family have a history of miscarriages or reproduction among close relatives? (Check both sides of family.)

Does your family have a history of genetic disease?

Did you have any problems getting pregnant? Did you use any conception aids?

How many children do you have?

- For each child, how did the delivery go?
    - method of delivery
    - length of delivery
    - gestational age
    - birth weight
    - health of the baby (heritable diseases/anatomical anomalies)

Have you ever miscarried and, if so, at what stage of pregnancy?

Were there any complications in any of your pregnancies (e.g., high blood pressure, diabetes)?

Were the labors unassisted or did you require forceps, vacuum, or a C-section?

How is your family support for this pregnancy?

Have you had contact with infectious disease during your current pregnancy?

How do you feel about becoming a mother? Would you choose to abort a fetus with a chromosomal abnormality?

Are you exposed to teratogen in your work or activities?

Do you drink or smoke?

Management

Counsel the patient about chromosomal abnormalities:

- Examples of chromosomal abnormalities include trisomy 21, trisomy 13, and open neural tube defects.
- The risk of chromosomal abnormalities increases with maternal age.
- Fetuses with more than one chromosomal abnormality (comorbid disease) are less viable.

Explain the protocols of prenatal screening:

- Screening is offered to mothers of all ages.
- Screening is available as an option, not an obligation.
- Screening must precede invasive testing, unless the patient is older than 40.

- Invasive testing is done only if the patient would terminate the pregnancy on a finding of abnormalities (abortion before week 20).

Explain the process of prenatal screening (see breakdown that follows).

TYPE OF SCREENING	TIMING AND PROCEDURES
First trimester screening	11 to 14 weeks
	Nuchal translucency US with serum free beta-hCG and pregnancy-associated plasma protein A (PAPP-A), depending on maternal age
Second trimester screening	16 to 18 weeks
	US for dating, growth and anatomical anomalies (open neural tube defect) with unconjugated estriol (E3), quantitative beta-hCG, and alpha fetoprotein (AFP)
Diagnostic testing	10 to 12 weeks
	Chorionic villi sampling (CVS)
	12–16 weeks
	Amniocentesis (results not available until weeks 17 to 20)

Explain the risks of chorionic villi sampling and amniocentesis:

- One percent result in miscarriage, infection, or bleeding.
- Not all defects are detected.

Discuss the implications of dilation and curettage (early diagnosis) versus dilation and evacuation (later diagnosis).

ROUTINE CARE

Counsel the patient about proper care for pregnancy in general:

- Several things should be avoided: irradiation (e.g., X-rays), smoking, alcohol, cat litter, drugs, hot tub/sauna, infection (e.g., rubella, HIV, chicken pox).
- Continue with sexual activity (if safe) and regular exercise.
- Supplement diet with calcium, iron, folic acid, and vitamin B_{12}. For women who do not consume an adequate diet: take a daily multivitamin.
- Aim for appropriate weight gain:
  - Most women gain 11 to 16 kg (25 to 35 lb).
  - Expect to gain 0.5 kg (1 lb) per month in the first half of pregnancy, and 0.5 kg (1 lb) per week in the second half of pregnancy.
- Danger signs include: bleeding, cramping (contraction), painful urination, vaginal itching/discharge/pain (vaginitis), and weight loss.

- Advanced maternal age has other risks: preeclampsia/eclampsia, chronic high blood pressure, obesity, diabetes, and fibroids.
- Begin routine pregnancy monitoring and investigations (see Table 19): schedule a visit every 4 weeks until week 28, then every 2 weeks until week 36, then every 1 week until delivery.

Table 19. ROUTINE PREGNANCY MONITORING AND INVESTIGATIONS

VISIT	ROUTINE MONITORING/INVESTIGATIONS
First visit	Serology: CBC, ferritin, blood type, varicella immunoglobulins, rubella immunoglobulins, syphilis, HIV, HBsAg
	Electrophoresis for women of African, Indian, Mediterranean descent (detect abnormal hemoglobin)
	Pelvic exam: Pap smear, culture for gonorrhea/chlamydia
	Document: weight, baseline blood pressure
28 weeks	Serology: CBC, RhoGAM to Rh- mothers
36 weeks	Rh antibody screen
	Group B *Streptococcus* screen

Case 40: Unwanted pregnancy counseling

A 24-year-old woman is pregnant, but she doesn't want to give birth to a child at this time in her life. Please take a history and discuss a management strategy with the patient.

Time: 10 minutes

History

The history should first confirm the pregnancy and then focus on the patient's reasons for not wanting the pregnancy.

HISTORY OF PRESENT ILLNESS

How do you know you are pregnant (e.g., pregnancy test, ultrasound)?

How many weeks pregnant are you? When was your last menstrual period?

FOCUSED QUESTIONS: UNWANTED PREGNANCY

What are your goals for this pregnancy (carry to term/abort/put up for adoption)?

Do you know your options?

What are your reasons for not wanting the baby?

- financial
- social situation: stability, life cycle (student, dependent adult)
- abuse or rape
- own medical situation
- concern about genetic risks

Are you aware of support services to help mothers?

What are your feelings regarding adoption? Abortion?

How much do you know about each?

How do your social supports feel (family, friends, partner)?

Is the father involved? How does the father feel?

What contraceptive method have you been using?

What method are you planning to use in the future?

Management

Counsel the patient about all the options for the pregnancy, including keeping the baby (see breakdown that follows).

OPTION	DETAILS
Therapeutic abortion: medical	If performed at < 8 weeks:
	• methotrexate + misoprostol
	• beta-hCG follow-up
	If performed at > 12 weeks:
	• prostoglandin intra-/extra-amniotically or IM
	Advantages: less invasive, private, immediate, patient autonomy
	Disadvantage: intensive and longer follow-up, risk of persistent pregnancy, cramping, heavy bleeding
Therapeutic abortion: surgical	If performed at < 10 weeks: vacuum aspiration
	If performed between 12–16 weeks: D&C
	If performed between 16–23 weeks: dilation with evacuation
	Advantages: only option for later gestational ages, permits fewer follow-ups
	Disadvantages: has a small risk of perforation, infection, sterility, cervix laceration, Asherman syndrome, retained product of conception, infection
Adoption	Multiple services/organizations available to offer financial, social, and emotional counseling and support
Keep the baby	Multiple services/organizations available to offer financial, social, and emotional counseling and support

Initiate investigations and follow-up care as required:

- Rh grouping of mother for prevention of Rh alloimmunization
- cervical cultures for STDs and bacterial vaginosis
- follow-up beta-hCG levels to ensure pregnancy has been aborted
- surgical consult if medical management fails

Case 41: Gestational hypertension, eclampsia

A woman who is 36 to 40 weeks pregnant presents with proteinuria and a blood pressure reading of 130/85 (from 110/65). Please take a history, provide a differential diagnosis, and outline a management plan.

Time: 10 minutes

History

HISTORY OF PRESENT ILLNESS

How long have you known you have high blood pressure? Did you have it before the pregnancy?

Are you on medication for high blood pressure?

How much weight have you gained during your pregnancy?

Have you had any infections during your pregnancy?

PAST MEDICAL HISTORY

Have you had other pregnancies? If so, were you diagnosed with preeclampsia?

Have you been diagnosed with any of the following?

- high blood pressure
- kidney disease
- type 2 diabetes
- obesity
- antiphospholipid antibody syndrome
- high cholesterol

Is there a history of preeclampsia in your family?

Do you use recreational drugs (cocaine, methamphetamine)?

Differential diagnosis

See Table 20.

Table 20. DIFFERENTIAL DIAGNOSIS OF GESTATIONAL HYPERTENSION/ECLAMPSIA

CONDITION	DIAGNOSTIC CRITERIA
Hypertension	DBP > 90 mmHg from at least 2 measurements
	SBP > 140 mmHg (does not strictly meet criteria for HTN, but monitor patient closely for developing DBP > 90 mmHg)
	Can be:
	• preexisting (resistant) or gestational
	• with or without proteinuria
	• with or without adverse effects (headache, kidney dysfunction, liver enzyme abnormalities, thrombocytopenia, etc.)
Severe hypertension	SBP > 160 mmHg or DBP > 110 mmHg with repeat confirmation in 15 minutes
Preeclampsia	Hypertension and proteinuria and/or nondependent edema at > 20 weeks pregnancy
	SBP increased 30 or DBP increased 15 or > 140/90
	Mild:
	• no neurological symptoms
	• none of the criteria for severe preeclampsia (see below)
	Severe:
	• onset before 34 weeks
	• heavy proteinuria: > 2+ or > 5 g/dL
	• BP > 160/100
	• complications with cardiovascular system (heart failure), kidneys (elevated serum creatinine, oliguria), liver (ascites, elevated liver enzyme and bilirubin), CNS (headache, visual disturbances, clonus)
Eclampsia	All of the criteria for preeclampsia plus seizure

Management

In all cases: if earlier than 34 weeks, administer corticosteroid therapy for pulmonary maturity before delivery.

Assess and treat the underlying condition (see breakdown that follows).

CONDITION	ASSESSMENT/TREATMENT
Preexisting HTN	**Assessment:** • baseline Cr, K and urinalysis and discontinue any ACE inhibitor or ARBs • urine for protein > 0.3 g/dL (> 30 mg/mmol) spot sample • if low risk for preeclampsia: urine dipstick • if suspicious for preeclampsia: 24 h protein, Cr **Treatment (nonsevere hypertension):** • antihypertensives: methyldopa, labetalol, other beta-blockers, nifedipine • without comorbidities: target SBP 130–155, DBP 80–105 • with comorbidities: target SBP 130–139, DBP 80–89
Mild preeclampsia	**Assessment:** • physical examination (mother) • CBC, electrolytes, urinalysis, PTT, INR, FDP, LFTs, 24 h urine, Cr clearance, protein • fetal evaluation: fetal heart rate, nonstress test (NST), biophysical profile (BPP) **Treatment:** • rest, left decubitus position • normal diet, no medication • monitoring of BP
Severe preeclampsia	Stabilize and deliver Admit: start IV, crossmatch blood, insert urine catheter, specify nothing by mouth (npo) Evaluate and monitor: • mother: vitals, input/output, deep tendon reflexes, urine protein, CBC, electrolytes, PTT, INR, FDP, LFTs, Cr clearance, urinalysis • fetus: continuous nonstress test (NST) Administer: • anticonvulsant: Mg sulfate ($MgSO_4$), 4 g IV push, then 2–4 g/h • antihypertensives: labetalol, nifedipine capsule, nifedipine PA tablets or hydralazine to target BPs < 160/110 Continue postpartum management for at least 24 h until stabilized
Eclampsia	Ensure ABCs Control seizures with $MgSO_4$ Monitor for complications: lung aspiration, acidosis, fracture Do not try to shorten or abolish initial convulsion: prevent injury to mother and maintain adequate oxygenation

Case 42: Abdominal pain and pregnancy

A 20-year-old pregnant woman presents with lower left quadrant (LLQ) pain. Please take a focused history, perform a physical exam, give a differential diagnosis, and propose investigations.

Time: 5 minutes

History

How many weeks pregnant are you?

Has there been any bleeding?

Have you felt the baby moving?

Have you had any contractions?

Have you been diagnosed with any of the following?

- high blood pressure
- preeclampsia
- previous abruption
- vascular disease

Have you had a recent trauma?

Do you use cocaine?

Physical examination

CATEGORY TO ASSESS	DETAILS
Vitals	BP sitting and supine, fetal heart rate
General condition	Pallor, diaphoresis, altered LOC
Abdomen	Inspection: surgical scars, shapes
	Palpation: pain, mass, rebound tenderness
	Percussion: fluid
	Auscultation: bowel sounds, fetal heart beat
Gynecology	Vaginal bleeding, cervical dilation

Differential diagnosis

Possible etiologies of abdominal pain during pregnancy include:

- ectopic pregnancy
- placenta abruption

- placenta previa
- abortion
- ovarian cyst (hyperreactio luteinalis)
- ovarian torsion

Investigations

Recommend:

- maternal: US, CBC, PTT, INR
- fetal: nonstress test (NST), heart rate, biophysical profile (BPP) by US

Case 43: Breast-feeding counseling

A 25-year-old woman who is pregnant has concerns about breast-feeding. Please take a history and discuss a management plan with her.

Time: 5 minutes

History

HISTORY OF PRESENT ILLNESS

What are your concerns about breast-feeding?

PAST MEDICAL HISTORY

Have you tried breast-feeding before? How did that go?

Do you have any of the following diseases?

- HIV/AIDS
- active or untreated TB
- regional herpes

What medications do you take?

Is chemotherapy or radiation therapy a concern for you?

Do you drink alcohol? How much, how often?

Do you use recreational drugs?

Management

Address the patient's specific concerns.

As appropriate, counsel the patient about the benefits of breast-feeding:

- Breast milk suits infants' immature GI tract, kidney, immune system, and metabolic demands.
- It provides excellent nutrition: 50% energy from fat, contains essential fatty acids, 90% absorption. Compared to cow's milk, breast milk has lower protein but more essential amino acids, higher whey content (easily digested protein), less casein, and it provides 50% iron absorption versus 10% absorption for cow's milk.
- It builds baby's immunity: IgA, macrophages, active lymphocytes, lysozyme; promotes growth of lactobacillus in GI tract.
- It is less allergenic.
- Babies still need supplements of vitamin D.
- Breast-feeding promotes bonding between mother and baby.

Counsel the patient about contraindications for breast-feeding:

- HIV/AIDS
- active or untreated TB
- regional herpes
- using alcohol/drugs
- chemo/radiation therapy

As appropriate, counsel the patient about alternatives to breast-feeding:

- formula brand: use an iron-fortified brand, and try to be consistent with one brand
- special formulas (if needed) for protein hypersensitivity, lactose intolerance, phenylketonuria (PKU)
- cow's milk:
  - no whole cow's milk in first year due to high renal protein loading, poor iron absorption
  - no reduced-fat milk (2% or less) in first 2 years: fat is required for neural development

Case 44: Cesarean section counseling

A 20-year-old woman is pregnant with her second child. She had a C-section with her first child due to fetal distress. She is concerned about having another C-section.

Time: 5 minutes

History

HISTORY OF PRESENT ILLNESS

How did your last pregnancy go?

Did you have any complications with your last pregnancy (e.g., hypertension, diabetes)?

Have your risk factors changed for this pregnancy?

Why was the decision made to have a C-section?

Why are you worried about second C-section (e.g., discomfort, scar, social support)?

Management

Counsel the patient about vaginal birth after cesarean (VBAC):

- Most women can have a successful vaginal delivery after a C-section, even after 2 C-sections.
- It is necessary to know the location of last uterine scar.
- Patients must deliver in a hospital with C-section capabilities.
- Procedure would involve:
  o admission as soon as labor starts
  o close monitoring of mother and baby
  o an attempt of vaginal delivery first
  o oxytocin for augmentation (prostaglandins not recommended)
  o C-section if required (still very safe)

Counsel the patient about contraindications for VBAC:

- inverted or classical C-section (risk of uterine rupture)
- previous uterine rupture
- placenta previa

Case 45: Birth control counseling

A 20-year-old woman requests birth control pills. Please take a history and counsel her.

Time: 5 minutes

History

HISTORY OF PRESENT ILLNESS

Have you used oral contraceptives before?

Are you looking for benefits other than contraception (e.g., heavy period control, acne control, control of irregular periods)?

Are you aware of other contraceptive methods?

Do you have a history of any of the following?

- breast cancer
- migraine with aura
- embolism, stroke, complicated valvular heart disease
- impaired liver function or liver tumor

Have you had a baby recently?

Is it possible you are pregnant now?

PAST MEDICAL HISTORY

Is there a history of high cholesterol in your family?

What is the pattern of your sexual activity?

Do you smoke?

Management

Answer the patient's questions.

Ensure the patient knows that her questions and your counsel are confidential.

Describe the anatomy and physiology of the reproductive cycle.

Counsel the patient about all contraceptive methods (see breakdown that follows).

METHOD	NOTES	FAILURE RATE	SIDE EFFECTS
Hormone			
Oral contraceptives	No STD protection Need to remember to take them	1% if taken as prescribed 3% compliance failure	Possible estrogen effects: worse migraines, increased body weight, higher blood pressure, aggravation of uterine fibromas, nausea Possible progesterone effects: depression, acne, more body hair, breast tenderness
Progesterone implant/ injection	No STD protection	0.01%	Possible progesterone effects: depression, acne, more body hair, breast tenderness
Barrier			
Condom	STD protection Some inconvenience	3%	None
Diaphragm	May provide STD protection Fitting required Jelly/cream required	6%	Possible increased UTIs Possible allergy
Vaginal sponge	May provide STD protection	6–9%	Possible toxic shock syndrome
Vaginal chemicals (foams, jelly, suppository)	May provide STD protection Some inconvenience	3%	Possible allergy
Other			
Physiologic (rhythm, coitus interruptus)	No STD protection Require significant motivation by couples, and regular menstrual cycles	4–5%	None
Surgical (tubal ligation, vasectomy)	No STD protection Irreversible	Vasectomy: 0.1%–0.2%	None
IUD	No STD protection Physician insertion and removal required	1%	Possible: cramping, midcycle bleeding, heavy periods, ectopic pregnancy, pelvic inflammatory disease perforation, expulsion

Since this patient is interested in oral contraceptives, describe how to use them:

- Take the first pill either today or the first Sunday after the start of bleeding, and take a pill daily. Use an alternate means of contraception for the first month of taking the pills.
- If you miss a pill, take 2 pills the next day. Use condoms or another prophylactic for the rest of that month.
- Vomiting or diarrhea can reduce the effectiveness of oral contraceptives: use alternate contraceptive methods.
- Oral contraceptives can interact with other medications, making them or the other medications less effective: check with your doctor each time you are put on new medications.

Case 46: Infertility

A 37-year-old woman, who has been married for 7 years, presents with infertility. Please obtain a focused history.

Time: 5 minutes

History

Interview both partners (the female and the male), and remember that infertility can be multifactorial.

HISTORY OF PRESENT ILLNESS (BOTH PARTNERS)

How long have you been trying to have a child?

How often have you been having intercourse?

At what point in the menstrual cycle are you having intercourse?

FOCUSED QUESTIONS: FEMALE

Have you ever been pregnant? If so, how many times?

Have you miscarried and, if so, at what stage of pregnancy?

Have you had problems getting pregnant before? Have you used any conception aids?

How many children do you have?

How old were you when you had your first period? (Or—as appropriate— when your breasts began to develop?)

How long is your usual cycle? How many days of bleeding are usual for you? How many pads or tampons do you usually use per day? Are there clots?

Has there been any change in your cycle?

Have you had a Pap smear before? What were the results of past Pap smears?

What gynecological procedures have you had (e.g., loop electrosurgical excision procedure, hysterectomy)?

Have you had any STDs?

Have you used contraception and, if so, what methods have you used?

Have you had any of the following?

- tubal disease, fibroids, endometriosis
- abdominal or pelvic surgery
- acne
- alopecia

Do you drink, smoke, or use recreational drugs?

What do you do for a living? (Assess for exposure to harmful chemicals.)

FOCUSED QUESTIONS: MALE

Have you had a pregnancy with any other sexual partners?

How is your sexual function?

What is the quality of your erections?

Do you have any difficulty ejaculating?

Have you had any previous investigations or procedures for fertility?

Do you take any medications?

Have you had previous chemotherapy or radiation therapy?

Have you had any of the following?

- mumps, TURP, hernia repair
- genital injuries (e.g., trauma, heat exposure)

Do you drink, smoke, or use recreational drugs?

What do you do for a living? (Assess for exposure to harmful chemicals.)

Case 47: Incontinence

A 75-year-old woman presents with incontinence. Please take a history and provide a differential diagnosis.

Time: 5 minutes

History

HISTORY OF PRESENT ILLNESS

When did the incontinence begin?

Does it involve gushes or leaking? Is the volume large or small?

How often does it happen?

Are you able to get to the bathroom?

Do you need to urinate at night?

Do you have a constant sense of bladder fullness?

What triggers the incontinence (e.g., laughing, coughing)?

Do any of the following apply to you?

- painful urination
- immobility
- recent infection
- sensory changes (e.g., tingling, numbness)
- fecal incontinence
- use of diuretics

PAST MEDICAL HISTORY

Have you been diagnosed with any of the following?

- type 2 diabetes
- urinary tract infections
- peripheral neuropathy
- spinal stenosis
- arthritis
- stroke
- dementia

Do you have children? If so, how many vaginal deliveries did you have?

Male patients: Have you had any prostate conditions or procedures (e.g., BPH, TURP)?

Differential diagnosis

Possible etiologies of incontinence, in either sex, include (mnemonic: **DIAPERS**):

- **d**elirium
- **i**nfection (UTI)
- **a**trophic vaginitis/urethritis
- **p**rostate enlargement/**p**harmaceuticals (diuretics, benzodiazepines, alcohol)/**p**sychological disorders
- **e**ndocrine disorders (hypercalcemia, DM, diabetes insipidus)
- **r**estricted mobility
- **s**tool impaction

Pediatrics

Case 48: Cough, asthma

A 2-year-old girl has developed a cough after being on antibiotics. Please obtain a history and provide a differential diagnosis.

Time: 5 minutes

History

HISTORY OF PRESENT ILLNESS

When does the coughing happen (e.g., after exertion, at night, in the morning)?

Are there any clear triggers for the coughing (e.g., smoke exposure, pet exposure, cold air)?

How does the cough sound?

Does she have shortness of breath? Wheezing? Does she turn blue?

Is she coughing anything up? What does it look like?

Does she have any of the following symptoms?

- cold symptoms
- runny nose
- fever
- weight loss
- sweats
- earache (pulling on ears)

Does she have any sick contacts (e.g., daycare)?

Does she seem to regurgitate food frequently or easily?

PAST MEDICAL HISTORY

Has your daughter ever been diagnosed with asthma?

Has she had any prescriptions for puffers or inhaled steroids? How did she respond to the treatment?

Has she ever been in the hospital for difficulty breathing?

Has anyone in your family been diagnosed with asthma or eczema?

Are her immunizations up to date?

Does anyone smoke at home?

Are there any pets at home?

Differential diagnosis

Possible etiologies of pediatric cough include:

- reactive airway disease
- croup
- URTI, bronchiolitis, bronchitis, pneumonia
- whooping cough
- foreign body
- environmental allergies (smoking, pets)
- cystic fibrosis
- bronchiectasis
- TB
- postnasal drip

Case 49: Diarrhea

A 1-year-old boy has had diarrhea for 6 months. Please obtain a history, provide a differential diagnosis, and recommend investigations.

Time: 5 minutes

History

The child seems to have chronic diarrhea (more than 2 to 3 weeks duration). The history should rule out celiac disease and other chronic etiologies.

HISTORY OF PRESENT ILLNESS

What is the diarrhea like (e.g., watery/solid, large/small volume, bloody, color)?

How many bowel movements does your son have a day?

Is the diarrhea constant? If it comes and goes, when does it happen? How long does it last?

Does your son have any fever, abdominal discomfort, or vomiting? If yes, do these symptoms happen before, during, or after a bowel movement?

Do you have any concerns about your son's development (e.g., sleep, growth, weight gain, reaching developmental milestones)?

Does your son seem pale?

When he cries, does he make tears? How many wet diapers does he have in a day?

What is your son eating? How much? How frequently?

Do you breast-feed him or give him formula?

Have there been any changes to his feeding pattern or his type of food?

Does he have any infectious contacts (e.g., daycare)?

PAST MEDICAL HISTORY

Is your son on any medications or antibiotics?

Does anyone in your family have similar symptoms?

Has anyone been diagnosed with celiac disease?

Have you traveled recently? Where?

Do you have pets at home?

Differential diagnosis

If the child exhibits failure to thrive, possible causes are:

- diet
- celiac disease
- milk protein allergy
- inflammatory bowel disease
- pancreas (e.g., cystic fibrosis)
- other: thyroid, Addison disease, IgA deficiency, AIDS, neoplasm

If the child is thriving, possible causes are:

- toddler's diarrhea
- infection (bacterial, parasites, *Clostridium difficile*)
- lactase deficiency

Investigations

INVESTIGATION CATEGORY	DETAILS
General chemistry	CBC, electrolytes, Cr, BUN
Growth	Height, weight, head circumference
Stools	C&S, ova and parasites (O&P), fecal occult blood test (FOBT), *C. diff*, fat content, pH, reducing substances
X-ray	Upper GI, barium enema
Mucosal disease	Endoscopy/mucosal biopsy
If failure to thrive	Alpha-1-antitrypsin, sweat chloride, thyroid function, HIV, albumen, electrolytes, CBC, ESR, protein

Case 50: Attention deficit hyperactivity disorder

A father comes to see you because he believes his child is hyperactive. Please obtain a history and discuss a management plan with the father.

Time: 5 minutes

History

HISTORY OF PRESENT ILLNESS

What is your child like when hyperactive? Please give some specific examples and situations.

When did this kind of behavior start?

How old is your child?

How is your child doing at home? At school? With friends?

Is your child experiencing any stress at home or at school?

Do you have any concerns about your child's development (e.g., growth, reaching developmental milestones)?

How is your child eating? Sleeping?

Is your child experiencing fevers, night sweats, or weight loss?

PAST MEDICAL HISTORY

Have you consulted a doctor about this before?

Has the child been prescribed any medication for this behavior? Did it make a difference?

Are your child's vaccinations up to date?

Are there any siblings or family members with similar behaviors?

Is there a possibility the child could be using street drugs or medications prescribed for someone else?

Management

If you suspect the behavior is related to stress (e.g., grief), reassure the father and counsel that it may take time to resolve. If the child is in school or daycare, suggest the father talk about the situation with the child's teachers or care staff.

If you suspect attention deficit/hyperactivity disorder (ADHD), counsel the father about the condition:

- ADHD can run in families.
- Chaotic environments at home, school, or daycare can make ADHD worse.
- ADHD usually arises before 7 years of age. It resolves for some people by early adolescence. It continues into adolescence for others (70% to 80%) and occasionally even into adulthood (15% to 20%).
- Psychostimulant medications (e.g., Ritalin) may control symptoms to a certain extent.
- Coping strategies at home and school are also crucial to managing ADHD. A psychologist can provide help with these.

Case 51: Speech delay

The parents of a 3-year-old girl are worried about her development. Her speech is far behind others in her age group. She only says "mom" and "dad." Compared to her older brother, she has been slower to achieve development milestones. Please obtain a history and give a differential diagnosis.

Time: 5 minutes

History

The history needs to begin with the child's symptoms and past medical history, and then focus on the mother's health during pregnancy.

HISTORY OF PRESENT ILLNESS

How long have you been concerned about your daughter's development?

How does she communicate with others? Is she interested in communicating?

What developmental milestones has she achieved? When did she achieve them?

Is she experiencing seizures?

Is she otherwise healthy?

PAST MEDICAL HISTORY

Has she had a history of any of the following?

- fevers
- ear infections
- meningitis
- trauma

Have you seen a doctor about your concerns before? Has she received any treatments as a result?

Do any diseases run in the family?

How is her older brother doing? When did he reach his developmental milestones?

FOCUSED QUESTIONS: MATERNAL HEALTH DURING PREGNANCY

Did you have any illnesses during pregnancy or breast-feeding?

Did you drink, smoke, take medications, or use recreational drugs while you were pregnant?

Was your daughter a full-term baby?

Did you have any complications during pregnancy or delivery?

Do you know her postdelivery Apgar scores?

Differential diagnosis

CATEGORY	POSSIBLE ETIOLOGY
Hearing impairment	Conductive or neurologic, genetic, congenital infections, meningitis, medications, otitis media
Cognitive disability	Pervasive developmental disorder, autism
Psychiatric	Selective mutism
Neurologic	Landau-Kleffner syndrome

Case 52: Speech impairment

A 6-year-old girl presents with dysphrasia. Please take a history and assess her status.

Time: 10 minutes

History

Take the history from the child's parent.

HISTORY OF PRESENT ILLNESS

When did you become concerned about your daughter's speech?

Which is her dominant hand?

What is her first language?

What grade is she in at school?

Has she been diagnosed with a learning disability?

Assessment

Interview the child during the assessment and focus on:

- fluency
- paraphrasic errors (e.g., *dook* for *book*, *table* for *desk*)
- comprehension: verbal/written
- writing skills

ASSESSMENT INTERVIEW

Can you hear me?

Are you right-handed or left-handed?

Please tell me about yourself (e.g., your favorite TV show, what you like to eat for supper, your favorite activity in school).

I'm going to point to some objects in the room. Can you tell me what they are?

Can you say these words after me? (Say a series of words and phrases.)

Please show me how you can write. (Give a simple topic such as: What is your favorite animal? What is your favorite food?)

Please read these words to me. (Write down, very legibly, some simple words such as *cat*, *red*, *desk*, *hat*.)

Case 53: Failure to thrive

An infant boy presents with failure to thrive. Please take a history and discuss a management strategy with the mother.

Time: 5 minutes

History

The history should first focus on the baby, and then on maternal health.

HISTORY OF PRESENT ILLNESS

How old is the baby?

Was he full term or premature?

How much did he weigh at birth? How much now? (Check height, weight, and head circumference against percentiles.)

How do you feed him (breast, bottle, formula)? How often?

Do you give him any supplements (e.g., iron, potassium, vitamin D, calcium)?

Do you have any concerns about the way he feeds (e.g., pauses during feeding)?

What are his stools like? How many bowel movements does he have per day?

How many wet diapers does he have per day?

Is he experiencing vomiting or diarrhea? If diarrhea, is there any blood? If vomiting, is it yellow-green (bile-stained)?

FOCUSED QUESTIONS: MATERNAL HEALTH

Do you have any diseases?

What medications are you taking?

Do you drink alcohol? How much, how often? Did you drink during pregnancy?

Do you smoke or use recreational drugs?

Management

If the mother is breast-feeding, counsel her to:

- supplement with iron by 6 months
- not smoke, drink, or use recreational drugs

Counsel her to stop breast-feeding:

- if she is on chemotherapy
- if she is taking certain medications (e.g., lithium, iodine-containing compounds, gold, anticancer drugs, immune suppressants)
- if she has an infection such as TB or HIV

If the mother is not breast-feeding, counsel her about:

- formula brand: use an iron-fortified brand, and try to be consistent with one brand
- special formulas (if needed) for protein hypersensitivity, lactose intolerance, phenylketonuria (PKU)
- cow's milk:
  - no whole cow's milk in first year due to high renal protein loading, poor iron absorption
  - no reduced-fat milk (2% or less) in first 2 years: fat is required for neural development
- vegetarian diet: not recommended in first 2 years of life

Advise the mother about an appropriate dietary schedule:

- 0 to 4 months: breast milk, formula
- 4 to 6 months: iron-enriched foods, cereals (rice cereals first), yellow-green veggies
- 6 to 9 months: pureed fruits/juice, meats, fish, poultry, egg, yogurt
- 9 to 12 months: finger foods, peeled fruits, cheese, cooked veggies (no raw veggies/hard fruits); no added salts, sugars, fats, seasoning

Counsel the mother to return in a few days to have the baby weighed, or to return sooner if she has concerns.

Case 54: Accidental ingestion

A mother phones your office in distress because her 18-month-old son has swallowed some antihypertensive medication. Please give her advice over the phone and outline a management plan for the emergency room.

Time: 5 minutes

Phone procedure

Get the mother's name, phone number, and address. Send an ambulance.

Inform the mother that an ambulance is coming.

If the child is unconscious, tell her to put the child in the recovery position, do a finger sweep, and protect the child's airways.

Tell her to check for breathing and a pulse.

- If not breathing, give 2 rescue breaths and check again.
- If no pulse, start cardiopulmonary resuscitation (CPR).

Tell her to bring the bottle of ingested medication to the hospital.

Ask:

- What was swallowed? How much (how much is left in the container)?
- When did you notice this had happened?
- Did it happen before or after a meal?
- What is the height, weight, and age of the child?
- Who found the child? What was the child doing? Unconscious? Confused? Complaining of discomfort? Vomiting?

Ask the mother to check for pills in the child's mouth and remove them. Ask her to remove any pills that may still be in the child's reach.

Ask the mother if she wants you to call poison control for further advice or if she can do it herself.

Inform emergency room staff of the incoming patient and clinical history.

Management (emergency room)

Ensure ABCs; monitor vitals; start IV hydration; insert nasogastric (NG) tube and Foley catheter as needed.

Admit for observation.

Consult with poison control; administer specific antidote if available.

Administer activated charcoal: 50–100 g (adult) or 30–50 g (child) via NG tube.

Initiate investigations:

- blood work: CBC, electrolytes, BUN, Cr, osmolality, LFTs, INR, PTT
- tox screen: urine

Case 55: Vomiting

A 6-week-old infant presents with a 3-day history of vomiting. Please take a history and recommend investigations.

Time: 5 minutes

History

HISTORY OF PRESENT ILLNESS

When did the vomiting start?

Is there a pattern to the vomiting (e.g., happens before or after a feeding)?

What does the vomit look like?

What is the vomiting like (e.g., projectile, not forceful)?

How is your baby otherwise (e.g., fussy, happy, hungry after vomiting)?

Have there been any changes to your baby's bowel movements?

How many wet diapers does your baby have per day?

Is your baby gaining weight and growing? (Check weight and height against percentiles.)

Do you have any concerns about your baby's development?

Have you changed your baby's diet recently?

How do you feed your baby (e.g., formula, breast)?

- If breast-feeding:
  - Have you changed your diet recently?
  - Are you on any medications?

Do you give your baby any supplements (e.g., iron, potassium, vitamin D, calcium)?

Investigations

Recommend:

- abdominal X-ray; US
- routine blood work

Case 56: Adolescent drug abuse

A mother comes to your office with her adolescent son, who is using drugs. She is seeking your advice on what to do. Please take a history and outline a management plan.

Time: 10 minutes

History

Take a history from the mother and the son separately. The same questions are useful in each interview and should cover:

- drugs being used
- living arrangements
- relationships (family, peers)
- school/work
- sexual activity
- suicide

HISTORY OF PRESENT ILLNESS

What substances are involved in the drug use?

What are the son's living arrangements (e.g., living with parents/others, people in the home)?

What are the son's relationships like?

- Does he have friends? Do his peers use drugs?
- How does he get along with his parents and other family members?
- What family issues are there?

Is the son attending school? What is school like for him? Does he have other regular activities (e.g., sports, work)?

Is he sexually active? Is he informed about safe sex, contraception, STDs? What is his sexual identity?

Is he having trouble with moods or suicidal thoughts (e.g., attempts, ideation, self-esteem, plans)?

Management

With the mother and son together, talk about:

- the effects of the drugs the son is using
- the importance of getting help (support groups, counseling)

Counsel them to involve the whole family in resolving the issue.

Emphasize the risk of alcohol, sexual activity, and other drugs.

Case 57: Epilepsy

A teenager with a history of epilepsy has been experiencing increased seizures. Please take a history and outline a management strategy.

Time: 5 minutes

History

The history should begin by assessing the severity of the seizures, and then focus on compliance with medications, and the use of alcohol and recreational drugs, as possible etiologies.

HISTORY OF PRESENT ILLNESS

How many seizures are you having per day?

How much have the seizures increased over what period of time?

How are the seizures affecting your day-to-day life (e.g., school life, work life, sleeping, driving, exercising)?

PAST MEDICAL HISTORY

What types of antiseizure medications are you taking? What dosages?

Are you taking them as prescribed?

What are your sleep patterns like?

How much and how often do you exercise?

Do you drink alcohol? How much, how often?

Do you use recreational drugs?

Are you experiencing any personal or interpersonal problems?

Management

Counsel the patient to address possible precipitating factors, such as compliance with medications, and cessation of alcohol or drug abuse.

Counsel the patient to keep a daily chart of the number, time, and circumstances of seizures.

Advise the patient of the possible need to change medications if the current one is not effective.

Remember to rule out and treat other possible causative factors:

- infections of CNS (bacterial/viral meningitis)
- neoplasms of CNS
- electrolyte imbalances (hyponatremia)
- endocrine disturbances (hypoparathyroidism, islet cell adenomas)

Advise the patient of the possible need to surgically eliminate the epileptic foci, which requires careful analysis of clinical factors, imaging, EEG, etc.

Case 58: Anemia

The parents of a 12-month-old boy have noted that their son seems pale. Please take a focused history and provide a differential diagnosis

Time: 5 minutes

History

The history needs to establish how certain the parents are of the baby's pallor, and then search for possible etiologies, including maternal health during pregnancy.

HISTORY OF PRESENT ILLNESS

When did you first notice that your son seemed pale?

Have you seen any changes in his color over time?

Does he have any of the following symptoms?

- appetite for unusual nonfood substances (pica)
- difficulty swallowing
- inflamed lips
- inflamed tongue
- fever
- signs of infection
- abdominal discomfort
- diarrhea

PAST MEDICAL HISTORY

Are you giving your son iron supplements?

What is his diet? How is he fed?

Is he gaining weight and growing? (Check weight, height, and head circumference against percentiles.)

Do you have any concerns about his development?

Has he had any illnesses? Has he been hospitalized?

Do you have other children? How are they doing?

Do any diseases run in your family?

What is your ethnicity?

FOCUSED QUESTIONS: MATERNAL HEALTH DURING PREGNANCY

Did you have any illnesses during pregnancy or breast-feeding?

Was your son a full-term baby?

Differential diagnosis

In children 3 to 18 months old, pediatric anemia is common.

After 18 months, consider the possibility of blood loss from:

- esophagitis
- peptic ulcer disease
- Meckel diverticulum
- inflammatory bowel disease
- celiac disease

Other conditions of importance in anemia include:

- thalassemia
- sickle cell disease
- infections

Case 59: Bloody diarrhea

A child has diarrhea with bloody stools. Please obtain a history.

Time: 10 minutes

History

When did the diarrhea start? When did the bloody stools start?

What is the volume of the stools? How much blood is there?

Has the child been experiencing any of the following?

- cough
- fever
- belly pain
- frequent bowel movement urgency (tenesmus)
- urine changes (e.g., low volume, blood in urine)
- skin rashes
- weight loss
- other bleeding (nose bleeds, easy bruising)

Has the child had any recent exposure to the following?

- animals, especially farm animals
- manure
- contaminated produce
- hamburgers

Has the child traveled recently?

Has the child eaten in a restaurant recently?

Have there been any recent changes to the child's diet?

Do any of the child's contacts have similar symptoms?

Case 60: Febrile seizure

A mother comes to your office because her 18-month-old daughter has had a seizure accompanied by a high fever. Please take a history and discuss a management plan with the mother.

Time: 5 minutes

History

The history needs to establish whether the child experienced a true seizure.

HISTORY OF PRESENT ILLNESS

When did the seizure happen?

What was the seizure like (e.g., localized, generalized)?

How long did it last?

Did the seizure result in any of the following for your daughter?

- bitten tongue
- fractures
- urinary incontinence
- trouble moving her body, difficulty speaking (neurological deficits)

Do any of the following apply to your daughter recently?

- fever (How high?)
- illness
- sleep deprivation
- electrolyte disturbances (problems with her sodium level)

PAST MEDICAL HISTORY

Is this the first time your daughter has had a seizure?

Do you have any concerns about her development (e.g., developmental milestones)?

Is your daughter taking any medications?

Are any of the following conditions or factors in her background? (Assess for epileptogenic risk.)

- head trauma
- surgery
- stroke
- central nervous system disease
- meningitis

Is there anyone in the family who has seizures?

FOCUSED QUESTIONS: MATERNAL HEALTH DURING PREGNANCY

Did you have any illnesses during pregnancy?

Did you drink, smoke, take medications, or use recreational drugs while you were pregnant?

Was your daughter a full-term baby?

Did you have any complications during pregnancy or delivery?

Do you know her postdelivery Apgar scores?

Management

Counsel the mother to:

- Administer acetaminophen.
- Give her daughter tepid sponge baths.
- Seek medical attention if she is concerned.

Educate her about seizures in children.

- Typical febrile seizures:
  - occur between 6 months and 6 years
  - accompany fever higher than 39°C (102.2°F) or a rapid rise in temperature
  - last less than 15 minutes, most less than 5 minutes
  - are generalized, symmetric, and involve the whole body
  - present with normal EEGs
  - don't recur within 24 hours
  - don't result in neurological deficits
- Risk of recurrence:
  - 33% generally
  - higher if onset occurred before 1 year old
  - usually don't occur after 6 years of age
- If a child has a complex seizure or a prior abnormal neurological exam:
  - risk of seizure recurrence is higher
  - risk of epilepsy is 5%

Case 61: Physical abuse

A parent brings an injured child to you. You suspect physical abuse. Please obtain a history, do a physical exam, and outline a management plan.

Time: 10 minutes

History

Interview the parents and the child separately. In each interview, obtain a detailed timeline and description of what happened. Document and date the information you obtain.

Some questions apply to both the child and the parents. Some focus on parent-specific issues and prenatal issues.

When the child is with one or both of the parents, assess their interaction.

HISTORY OF PRESENT ILLNESS: CHILD AND PARENTS SEPARATELY

What, where, when, why, and how did this happen to the child?

Who was at home at the time (e.g., what adults, other children)?

Who lives at home?

Does the child go to daycare or school? How is that going?

What activities does the child engage in?

FOCUSED QUESTIONS: PARENTS

Do you have any concerns about your child's development (e.g., developmental milestones, physical disability, hyperactivity, difficulty with discipline)?

Have you had any concerns about bonding with your child?

What happens when the child cries?

What is the child's diet like?

Are the child's immunizations up to date?

Are you experiencing stress in your life (e.g., financial stress, relationship stress)?

Do you drink alcohol? How much, how often?

Do you use recreational drugs?

Is there physical abuse among other household members?

Do any of the following apply to you?

- physically abused as children
- illnesses
- psychiatric issues

Was this child a planned pregnancy?

Did you have any illnesses during pregnancy?

Did you drink, smoke, take medications, or use recreational drugs while you were pregnant?

Was the child a full-term baby?

Did you have any complications during pregnancy or delivery?

Do you know the child's postdelivery Apgar scores?

Physical exam

Assess whether the injury on exam correlates with the history provided.

Look for signs of unexplained injuries:

- lash marks, loop marks, restraint marks
- cigarette burns
- bruises in atypical places
- bite marks more than 3 cm wide (indicates adult inflicted)
- retinal hemorrhages
- posterior fractures
- venereal disease in prepubescent children
- multiple injuries of different ages
- symmetrical, instrument-shaped bruising above waist

Assess:

- signs of neglect (dirty, malnourished, failure to thrive, chronic infections)
- social isolation/apathy

Management

As appropriate:

- Document your findings and report them to the appropriate authorities (e.g., family and children's services).
- Admit the child to hospital for further workup.

Case 62: Neonatal jaundice

An infant girl presents with jaundice 48 hours after birth. Please obtain a history from the mother and provide a differential diagnosis.

Time: 5 minutes

History

The history should begin with questions about prenatal issues, and then focus on the infant.

HISTORY OF PRESENT ILLNESS: PRENATAL ISSUES

During your pregnancy and delivery, did you have any of the following?

- intrauterine infection or neonatal sepsis
- early rupture of membranes
- thyroid issues

Did you smoke or drink alcohol while you were pregnant?

What medications did you take (e.g., for thyroid issues, over-the-counter medications)?

How did you deliver this baby (vaginally or by C-section)? Were there any complications?

Are there any genetic diseases in your family?

What is your blood type and Rh status? What is the father's?

Do you have any other children with jaundice?

FOCUSED QUESTIONS: INFANT

Is this your first baby?

Was the delivery on time? If not, how many days before or after your due date did it occur?

Did the baby have any trauma from the delivery (e.g., scalp bruising)?

What time was the baby born? Did the jaundice start within the first 24 hours?

Do you know the baby's postdelivery Apgar scores?

How long did the baby stay in the hospital?

How is the baby feeding?

Does the baby have wet diapers?

What are the baby's stools like?

What is the baby's sleep pattern?

Did the baby pass meconium (have her first bowel movement) before delivery?

Did the baby have any tests done at birth?

Did the baby receive light therapy?

Differential diagnosis

Note:

- In neonates, unconjugated (indirect) hyperbilirubinemia is predominant.
- Conjugated (direct) hyperbilirubinemia due to intra- or extrahepatic biliary obstruction is rare.
- Rh hemolysis rarely occurs in a first baby, but ABO hemolysis does.
- ABO hemolysis is mostly seen in a baby with AB type blood and mother with O blood type.

TYPE	SIGNS
Physiologic jaundice	Appears > 24 hours of age
	Peaks by day 3
	Resolves by week 1
Pathologic	Appears < 24 hours of age
	Lasts > 1 week

If the jaundice lasts more than 3 weeks, rule out:

- breast milk jaundice
- hypothyroidism
- hepatitis
- conjugation dysfunction, metabolic
- impaired excretion

If it occurs within the first 24 hours, always consider pathologic etiology.

- Causes of bilirubin overproduction:
  - hemolysis (ABO/Rh incompatibility, glucose 6 phosphate deficiency, hereditary spherocytosis)
  - hemorrhage (scalp bruising/hematoma)
  - polycythemia (intrauterine growth restriction)
- Causes of decreased hepatic processing:
  - sepsis (impaired liver function)
  - prematurity (insufficient liver enzymes)
  - Crigler-Najjar syndrome (congenital absence of liver enzyme)
  - breast-feeding (inhibits liver enzymes)
  - hypothyroidism, Down syndrome (low or absent liver enzymes)

Case 63: Delayed passage of meconium

A newborn baby has delayed passage of meconium. Please provide a differential diagnosis and outline a management plan, including investigations.

Time: 5 minutes

Differential diagnosis

Possible etiologies of delayed passage of meconium include:

- Hirschsprung disease
- ileal atresia
- cystic fibrosis
- functional immaturity of the colon
- colon atresia
- extrinsic compression of the distal bowel by a mass lesion
- mesenteric cyst
- paralytic ileus
- sepsis

Management

Observe the infant for meconium passage.

If delayed more than 48 hours, do a barium enema to look for Hirschsprung disease and consult pediatric surgery.

Consider: US or CT scan, sweat chloride test.

Case 64: Sexual abuse

A 6-year-old girl has pain on micturition. You suspect sexual abuse. Please obtain a history from the mother and outline a strategy for management.

Time: 5 minutes

History

Child victims of sexual abuse may present with physical findings including anogenital problems, enuresis, or encopresis. Behavioral changes may involve sexual acting out, aggression, depression, eating disturbances, and regression.

HISTORY OF PRESENT ILLNESS

Is this your daughter's first urinary tract infection? If not, how frequent have they been? How have they been treated?

When did this problem begin?

Do any of the following conditions apply to your daughter?

- abdominal pain
- fever
- uncontrolled urination
- defecating in places other than the toilet

PAST MEDICAL HISTORY

Has your daughter been left with a male relative or friend (e.g., father, brother, uncle, neighbor)?

Do you have suspicions about anyone behaving improperly with your daughter?

Is there any drug or alcohol abuse at home?

Has a male relative or friend ever abused you, your child, or other children?

Do you have any concerns about your daughter in the following areas?

- sexual knowledge
- depression or anxiety
- self-esteem
- substance use
- eating disorder
- relationships with others

Are there other children at home?

Management

Arrange to interview the child separately from the mother.

Because physical exam findings of most child victims of sexual abuse are often within normal limits or nonspecific, getting a statement from the child is very important. Document and date the information you obtain.

Contact authorities as appropriate (police, child protection services).

Recommend support measures for the family (e.g., counseling, support groups).

Consider referring the child to a child psychiatrist.

Consider admitting the child to hospital.

Case 65: Low birth weight

A 45-year-old woman has delivered a low-birth-weight baby. Please obtain a focused history, and provide a differential diagnosis that lists complications.

Time: 5 minutes

History

The history should focus on the cause of the low birth weight and on possible complications resulting from it.

HISTORY OF PRESENT ILLNESS

Was the delivery on time? If not, how many days before or after your due date did it occur?

Did you have any complications during the delivery?

Did you have any diseases or issues during pregnancy (e.g., infections, fever, hepatitis)? Did you have regular prenatal checkups?

Did you smoke, use alcohol, or take medications or recreational drugs while you were pregnant?

How much weight did you gain during pregnancy?

Did you have any ultrasound exams during pregnancy? When and what were the results?

Do you have other children? How are they doing?

Are there any genetic conditions in the family?

What is your blood type and Rh status? What is the father's?

Is your baby symmetrically small or asymmetrically small?

How is the baby's tone? How is the baby feeding?

Do you know the baby's postdelivery Apgar scores?

How old are you? What is your ethnicity? Are you (the parents) of small stature?

Differential diagnosis

Possible etiologies for low birth weight include:

- intrauterine growth retardation
- congenital anomalies
- intrauterine exposure to alcohol or tobacco
- prematurity

Case 66: Acne

A 15-year-old girl wants advice about her acne. Please take a history and discuss a management plan with her.

Time: 5 minutes

History

HISTORY OF PRESENT ILLNESS

How long have you had acne?

Where is the acne (e.g., face, neck, back, chest)?

Do you have any pain, infection, or scarring with the acne?

Do you have any of the following symptoms? (Assess for polycystic ovarian syndrome.)

- excess body hair (e.g., face, chest)
- areas of dark-colored skin (e.g., armpits, groin, neck)

PAST MEDICAL HISTORY

Are you trying any treatments for the acne now? Have you tried any in the past?

What do you do to clean the affected skin?

How old were you when you had your first period? (Or—as appropriate—when your breasts began to develop?)

How long is your usual cycle? How many days of bleeding are usual for you? How many pads or tampons do you usually use per day? Are there clots?

Has there been any change in your cycle?

Do you use birth control pills?

Has the acne affected your social life?

Management

Counsel the patient that acne is common: 75% of teenagers are affected, and adults can be affected, too.

Explain that 2 kinds of treatment are available: topical and oral.

Topical therapies include:

- retinoids
- antimicrobials (benzoyl peroxide, clindamycin)
- salicylic acid
- steroid injection for severe painful episodes

Oral therapies include:

- oral antibiotics
- oral contraceptives (for female patients)
- Accutane for severe cases
  - Because of the risk of birth defects, female patients must use birth control while taking Accutane.
  - Patients should never share this medication with female friends.
  - Patients need liver function tests: first to establish a baseline and then to monitor (at 2 weeks after baseline and then monthly).

Preventive medicine and community health

Case 67: Sexual assault

A patient has been sexually assaulted. Please take a history.

Time: 5 minutes

History

Be sympathetic and respectful as you take the history.

HISTORY OF PRESENT ILLNESS

Who assaulted you?

How many assailants were there?

When did the assault happen?

Did penetration occur (anal, vaginal, oral)?

Did any physical assault or use of weapons occur?

What did you do after the assault (e.g., urinate, defecate, change clothes, shower, douche, etc.)?

When was your last voluntary intercourse?

PAST MEDICAL HISTORY

Do you have any chronic health problems?

Have you had any surgeries?

Do you have any allergies?

What medications do you take?

Have you been vaccinated against hepatitis B?

FOCUSED QUESTIONS (FEMALE PATIENTS): GYNECOLOGICAL HISTORY

When was your last menstrual period?

Have you ever been pregnant? If so, how many times (including full-term pregnancies, miscarriages, therapeutic abortions)?

Do you use contraception and, if so, what method are you using now?

Management

Ensure ABCs and manage injuries.

Ensure the patient is not left alone and has ongoing emotional support.

Set aside sufficient time for a physical exam (usually 1.5 hours).

Obtain consent for the physical exam and treatment, evidence collection, and disclosure to police. Notify police as soon as consent has been obtained.

Use a sexual assault kit and sexual assault protocol to ensure uniformity and completeness of the physical exam and evidence collection.

Maintain the chain of evidence: label samples immediately, pass them directly to police without leaving them unattended.

Address HIV prophylaxis, hepatitis B immunization/prophylaxis, tetanus immunization, and pregnancy.

Note that the patient may also be at risk of suicide and other forms of assault. Develop an exit plan that keeps the patient safe. Use community services (for shelter, emergency services, and legal counsel) as required.

As required, refer the patient to social workers or agencies that support victims of domestic violence.

Case 68: Breast health

A 30-year-old woman wants to learn how to do a breast self-exam. Please counsel her.

Time: 5 minutes

Management

Ask if there are specific concerns the patient would like to address.

Explain the breast self-exam technique (see breakdown that follows). Use your own body to demonstrate procedures as appropriate.

SELF-EXAM CATEGORY	DETAILS
Timing	If menstruating: check monthly after age 20 at the same time every menstrual cycle (e.g., 2–3 days after period ends); have an exam by a physician every 1–2 years before age 40
	If no longer menstruating: check the same day every month (e.g., the first day of each month); have an exam by a physician every year
Visual inspection (use mirror as appropriate)	
Breasts in general	Check for changes in size, symmetry
Nipple and areola	Check for changes in shape, position, color, symmetry, smoothness
	Check for local retractions
Skin	Check for changes in color, texture, venous pattern
	Check for ulceration, dimpling, swelling
Palpation	
Breasts	Use a systematic technique (clock or quadrant exam); include the tail of Spence and areola
	Check for changes in texture, symmetry, tenderness
	Check for masses (mobility, size)
	Gently squeeze the nipple to check for discharge
Lymph nodes	Check the entire axillary area for enlarged nodes

Case 69: Breast cancer

A 30-year-old woman is seeking advice because her mother and 2 sisters have all had breast cancer. Please take a history, recommend appropriate investigations, and discuss a management plan with her.

Time: 5 minutes

History

HISTORY OF PRESENT ILLNESS

Have you noticed any abnormalities or changes in your breasts?

PAST MEDICAL HISTORY

Have you been diagnosed with any of the following?

- breast cancer
- benign breast diseases
- obesity

Have you ever had an operation on your breasts or previous investigation of a breast lump or lesion?

Have you had any radiation to your chest or axillae?

What is your history with oral contraceptives and hormone replacement therapy?

How old were your family members when diagnosed with breast cancer? Was the cancer in one breast or both? What kind of treatment did they require?

Do you have children? If so, did you breast-feed them?

Do you drink or smoke?

Investigations

Recommend:

- breast exam
- mammogram

Management

Counsel the patient about her risk factors for breast cancer, depending on her history. (See Table 21 for information on all risk factors.)

Table 21. RISK FACTORS FOR BREAST CANCER

FACTOR CATEGORY	FACTOR
Nonmodifiable	Genetic: family history of breast cancer (having 1 first-degree relative with breast cancer doubles risk, having 2 first-degree relatives with breast cancer triples risk)
	Sex: females > males
	Menarche < age 12; menopause > age 55
	Prior history of breast cancer
	History of some benign breast diseases: moderate/floral hyperplasia, atypical hyperplasia, sclerosing adenosis, papilloma
Modifiable	Alcohol
	Smoking
	Obesity
	Oral contraceptive use (debated) or hormone replacement therapy for > 5 years (unopposed estrogen)
	Nulliparity, no lactation
	Late age of first pregnancy
	Radiation exposure

Counsel her that early diagnosis and management are key to a cure. Survival rates depend on how far the cancer has spread once detected:

- localized to breast: 80% 5-year survival
- localized to breast with estrogen receptor (ER) positivity: 90% 5-year survival
- positive lymph nodes: 50% 5-year survival, 25% 10-year survival

Counsel her to do monthly breast self-exams and get appropriate physician exams (see Case 68). She should also get appropriate regular mammograms. Recommendations may vary by jurisdiction. The current Canadian recommendations for average risk women are given in the breakdown that follows. For high risk women (women who have a personal or family history of breast cancer, BRCA1 or BRCA2 gene mutation, or prior chest wall radiation), screening recommendations may also vary by jurisdiction; often, screening involves annual mammography with or without breast MRI.

AGE	RECOMMENDED MAMMOGRAM SCREENING
40–49	Routine screening not recommended
50–69	Every 2–3 years
70–74	Every 2–3 years
75 and older	Insufficient data

Case 70: Erectile dysfunction

A 30-year-old man is experiencing erectile dysfunction. Please take a history, provide a differential diagnosis, and recommend investigations.

Time: 5 minutes

History

The history needs to establish what the patient means by erectile dysfunction.

HISTORY OF PRESENT ILLNESS

When did the problem start?

What is the problem with sexual function (e.g., arousal, maintaining erection, premature ejaculation, difficulty with orgasm)?

Is the problem constant or intermittent?

Does anything make the problem better or worse?

Do you have any current sexual partners?

What is the status of your relationship with your sexual partner(s) (e.g., long-term relationships, new relationships)?

Do you experience the problem when you masturbate?

Do you have early morning erections?

PAST MEDICAL HISTORY

Do any of the following conditions or factors apply to you?

- serious illness (e.g., diabetes, hypertension, atherosclerosis)
- trauma or surgery in the groin
- spinal injury
- prostatectomy, or other prostate conditions or procedures
- colorectal surgery
- radiation therapy
- changes in the distribution of body hair or fat, or in your voice

What medications do you take?

Do you use contraception? If so, what form?

Do any diseases run in your family?

Do you know of family members who have experienced erectile dysfunction?

What is your sexual orientation?

Do you drink, smoke, or use recreational drugs?

Differential diagnosis

ETIOLOGY	TYPICAL PRESENTATION
Psychological —50% of patients	Young age
	Intermittent symptoms
	No risk factors
	Nocturnal penile tumescence
	Ability to self-stimulate
Organic (nonpsychological) —50% of patients	> 50 years old
	No nocturnal penile tumescence
	Risk factors present:
	• endocrine: DM, gonadal dysfunction, pituitary dysfunction
	• cardiovascular: HTN, atherosclerosis
	• neurologic: sacral plexus problems, spinal cord disease/injury
	• iatrogenic: antihypertensives, radiation, surgery
	• penile: postpriapism, Peyronie disease

Investigations

Recommend, as appropriate:

- serum tests: testosterone, FSH, LH, prolactin, glucose, cholesterol

Consider recommending, depending on the specific circumstances:

- nocturnal penile tumescence monitor
- Doppler, penile blood pressure
- angiography, cavernosography, penile injection
- sacral nerve reflex latency time

Case 71: STD

A 28-year-old man presents with penile discharge. Please obtain a history, perform a physical exam, provide a differential diagnosis, and recommend investigations.

Time: 10 minutes

History

HISTORY OF PRESENT ILLNESS

How long have you had this problem?

Have you had recent unprotected sex? If so, when? (Assess incubation period.)

Do you have sexual partners with similar complaints (e.g., rectal or vaginal discharge)?

What is the color and odor of the discharge? How much is there? How often does it occur?

Do you have any of the following symptoms?

- penile pain or itchiness
- pain with urination (Confirm timing of pain: beginning, during, or end of urination.)
- swelling or pain in your joints or bones
- burning, gritty, or red eyes
- anal or rectal pain, bleeding, diarrhea, mouth pain, sore throat
- fever, swollen lymph nodes, weight loss
- skin rash, ulcer, penile warts, or herpes

PAST MEDICAL HISTORY

Have you had this kind of problem before?

Have you been diagnosed with or treated for any STDs?

Have you ever been diagnosed with hepatitis, tuberculosis, HIV, or other diseases?

Are you taking any medications? Have you changed any of your medications recently?

What is your sexual orientation?

How many sexual partners have you had in the last 6 months?

Do you have anal, vaginal, or oral sex?

Do you drink, smoke, or use recreational drugs?

Physical exam

Inspect external genitalia, including anus, for wounds, ulcers, warts, rash, other lesions, and obvious discharge.

Inspect oropharynx for lesions if the patient has a history of oral sex.

Palpate inguinal lymph nodes for adenopathy.

Differential diagnosis

FINDING	POSSIBLE ETIOLOGY
Discharge/discomfort	Chlamydia, gonorrhea, *Trichomonas*, *E. coli*
Ulcers	Syphilis, herpes, lymphogranuloma venereum (LGV), chancroid
Lesions	Human papilloma virus (HPV), carcinoma

Investigations

Recommend:

- CBC, urinalysis, urine C&S
- swabs for culture
- HBsAg, HBeAg, HIV, VDRL, RPR, CMV, HBcAg, anti-HCV

Case 72: Immunizations

A new immigrant mother wants information about immunizing her baby. Please take a history and discuss a management plan with her.

Time: 5 minutes

History

Which country are you from?

What vaccines has your baby had?

Is your baby currently ill?

Has your baby had high fever, meningitis, or neurological diseases?

Does your baby have any allergies (eggs, neomycin)? Has your baby had any reaction to previous vaccines?

What do you know about vaccinations?

Do you have any questions or concerns about vaccinations?

Management

Provide general information about vaccines and childhood diseases, as appropriate:

- A vaccine is a biological product that can cause a specific immune response when given to a healthy person. This immune response will protect the person from getting a specific disease.
- Vaccines are available for the 6 main killers of children worldwide:
  - measles
  - whooping cough (pertussis)
  - tetanus
  - polio
  - TB
  - diphtheria
- They are also available for other important diseases, including hepatitis, influenza, mumps, and rubella.
- Possible adverse reactions to a vaccine include local symptoms such as induration and tenderness at the site of injection. Systemic reactions include fever, rash, and crying. Allergic complications may include hives, stuffy or runny nose, and anaphylaxis.
- Contraindications to vaccination include:
  - allergies to vaccine components
  - severe illness with or without fever
  - immunodeficiency
  - unstable neurological disease
- Children are immunized on a schedule (see Table 22). Note that the schedule may vary from jurisdiction to jurisdiction.

Table 22. TYPICAL IMMUNIZATION SCHEDULE FOR CHILDREN*

AGE	DTaP-IPV-Hib	DTaP-IPV	MMR	HepB	DTaP	VZ	MENIN	PNEU	INFL**
2 mo	X						X	X	
4 mo	X						X	X	
6 mo	X						X	X	X
1 y			X			X			X
18 mo	X							X	X
4.5 y		X	X			X			

(Continued)

Table 22. (*Continued*)

AGE	DTaP-IPV-Hib	DTaP-IPV	MMR	HepB	DTaP	VZ	MENIN	PNEU	INFL**
Gr 5				X		X			
Gr 9					X				

* varies by jurisdiction: refer to local recommendations

** children 6–23 months should receive yearly

Legend

DTaP-IPV diphtheria, tetanus, acellular pertussis, polio

Hib hemophilus influenza B

MMR measles, mumps, rubella

HepB hepatitis B

DTaP diphtheria, tetanus, pertussis

VZ varicella zoster

Menin meningococcal C conjugate

Pneu pneumococcal conjugate

Infl influenza

Case 73: Falls

An elderly man has made an appointment because he has experienced 2 falls. The man's son has accompanied him to the appointment, and is concerned about injury to his father from falling and about his father's mobility. Please take a history, provide a differential diagnosis, and recommend investigations.

Time: 5 minutes

History

While taking the history, keep in mind that falls in the elderly can be multifactorial.

HISTORY OF PRESENT ILLNESS

How many times have you fallen?

When did the problem start? When was the last time you fell?

Are there any clear triggers for the problem (e.g., getting up from bed, turning, reaching, alcohol use)?

Do any environmental factors contribute to the problem (e.g., shoes, flooring, steps, lighting)?

During a fall, do you experience nausea or vomiting, or incontinence?

Do any of the following apply to you?

- weakness, sudden losses in strength
- sensations in limbs (tingling)

- use of mobility aids or other aids for activities of daily living
- past injuries (hip or limb fractures, head injury)
- recent infection
- recent change in medications or medication dose

What do you usually eat for breakfast, lunch, and supper? (Assess nutritional status.)

PAST MEDICAL HISTORY

Have you been diagnosed with any of the following?

- coronary artery disease
- atrial fibrillation
- arrhythmia
- stroke
- vision impairment
- arthritis
- peripheral neuropathy
- type 2 diabetes
- hypotension
- adrenal insufficiency
- seizures

What medications do you take (e.g., anticoagulants, diuretics, beta-blockers, antiarrhythmics, benzodiazepine)?

Do you drink alcohol? How much, how often?

Do you have a history of alcohol abuse?

Differential diagnosis

CATEGORY	POSSIBLE ETIOLOGY
Cardiac disorder	Arrhythmia, postural hypotension, valvular disease
Autonomic neuropathy	Type 2 diabetes
Discoordination	Parkinson disease, stroke, mass effect from subdural hemorrhage (SDH)
Delirium	Medications, infection, electrolyte imbalance, endocrinopathy
Dizziness	Vertigo, basilar stroke
Immobility/frailty	Weakness, poor reaction time, sensory impairment, anemia
Environmental factors	Loose rugs, poor footwear, wet floors

Investigations

Take the patient's blood pressure, both sitting and standing, and in both arms each time.

Recommend:

- CBC, electrolytes, Cr, PTT, INR
- EKG, 24 h Holter
- X-ray of potential fractured limbs
- carotid Doppler
- CT of head if concerned about intracranial hemorrhage or subdural hematoma (SDH)

Case 74: Risks of HIV for health care workers

A nurse has had a needle-stick injury from a source patient who was HBsAg positive and HIV negative. Please take a history and discuss a management plan with the patient.

Time: 5 minutes

History

What were the circumstances of the injury: where, when, with what (injection, bore, etc.)?

Did you have contact with feces, urine, or saliva?

Were universal precautions taken (gloves, gown, eye protection, etc.)?

What is your vaccination history for hepatitis (number of shots, titer checks)?

Management

Provide general information about the risk of contracting hepatitis and HIV from needle-stick injuries:

- Risk of contracting hepatitis B from a needle-stick injury with contaminated blood is 62%; risk of contracting hepatitis C, approximately 0.5%.
- Every health care worker should be vaccinated and have titers checked.
- Risk of contracting HIV from a needle-stick injury with contaminated blood is 0.3%. Taking zidovudine can reduce the risk of transmission by 80%.

- Universal precautions are essential.
- Use condoms (safe sex) after a needle-stick injury.

Describe procedures for infection control:

- Handle sharps, objects, and equipment with care.
- Do not recap, bend, break, or remove needles from syringes.
- Discard sharps in sharps containers.
- Specimen-collection protocol should be observed.
- Gloves should be worn for contact with blood, body fluids, broken skin, or mucus membranes.
- Change gloves after each patient contact.
- Wash hands after contact with blood or body fluids.
- Wear protective clothing (e.g., gowns, goggles, mask).
- Report needle-stick injuries to your health office and complete accident forms/protocol.

Counsel the patient about next steps (see breakdown that follows, which outlines treatment for all HBV/HIV eventualities).

STATUS OF SOURCE PATIENT	TREATMENT FOR HEALTH CARE WORKER
HBV+	If vaccinated for HBV, no treatment necessary. Monitor 3–6 months.
	If not vaccinated, give HBIg 0.06 mL/kg immediately. Start vaccine at 0, 1, 6 months, then monitor 0, 3, 6 months. (Note: HBIg is ideally given within 14 days of exposure, but it is still effective if given within 30 days.)
HBV–	No treatment necessary.
HIV+	Advise worker to use barrier protection for sex.
	Start combined therapy ASAP:
	• 3TC 150 mg bid for 4 wk
	• AZT 200 mg tid for 4 wk
	• indinavir (IDV) 800 mg tid for 4 wk
	Check latest guidelines.
HIV–	A small risk of infection exists, because source patient may test negative while incubating the virus.
	Advise worker to use barrier protection for sex.
	Follow up with HIV test in 3–6 months.

Case 75: Intimate-partner violence

A woman has been physically assaulted by her partner. Please take a history and outline a management plan.

Time: 10 minutes

History

Know the risk factors for intimate partner violence:

- Women are most at risk if they are pregnant, disabled, or 18 to 24 years of age.
- Male batterers: 80% were abused as children and/or witnessed violence in the home as children.
- Battered women: 67% witnessed their mothers being abused.
- Alcohol may contribute to violence but is not the cause.
- Violent partners are not always violent outside the home.
- Rigid definitions of male and female roles are common in abusive relationships, but either partner can be a victim of abuse.
- Abuse can occur in same-sex relationships.
- Abusive partners may feel excessive jealousy, lack trust for their partner or others, and have an inability to express or control anger.

HISTORY OF PRESENT ILLNESS

Has your partner hit you before? If so, how often does this happen?

In what ways is your partner abusive (e.g., physically, sexually, emotionally)?

Are there children in the home? Do they witness the abuse? Are they also victims of abuse?

Were you abused, or did you witness abuse, as a child?

Does your family have financial concerns?

Are you or your partner under stress?

Do you or your partner abuse alcohol or drugs? If so, what type, quantity, and frequency?

How do you solve differences with your partner?

Do you have anyone to turn to for help?

Do you have somewhere to go if you need to leave the home?

Have you ever been involved with a shelter or other support group?

Are you financially dependent on your abusive partner?

Have the police ever been involved in this problem?

Management

Cases of intimate-partner violence require the following steps: recognition, evaluation, documentation, and referral.

RECOGNITION

Suspect abuse if the patient presents with:

- serious bleeding injury to trunk, or with bruises, welts, burns, dislocated or broken bones, torn ligaments, perforated eardrums, dental injuries, injuries of various ages
- frequent visits for nonspecific complaints
- psychological difficulties: anxiety, depression, suicidal thoughts, drug/alcohol abuse

EVALUATION

Interview the victim alone, and use nonjudgmental but direct questions.

Reinforce that assault is a crime: don't blame the victim.

Ask about the safety of children or other members of the household.

DOCUMENTATION

Describe physical trauma and photograph injuries.

Describe psychological symptoms. Quote the patient directly.

REFERRAL

Refer the patient to social services agencies.

Ensure the patient has a safe place to go after disclosure (e.g., family, friend, shelter).

Case 76: Tuberculosis

A woman who has recently emigrated has had a chest X-ray as part of a screening process for her work. The X-ray is abnormal. Please take a history and provide a differential diagnosis.

Time: 5 minutes

History

HISTORY OF PRESENT ILLNESS

Before this most recent X-ray, when was the last time you had a chest X-ray? What were the results?

Do you cough? What is the sputum like (e.g., bloody, pink, putrid, puss-filled, copious)?

Do any of the following apply to you?

- bone pain
- headache
- weight loss (How much over how long?)
- recent contact with TB
- recent contact with bird feces (Assess for histoplasmosis, coccidiomycosis.)
- fever
- sputum production
- shortness of breath

PAST MEDICAL HISTORY

Have you been diagnosed with any of the following?

- cancer (e.g., testicle, breast, colon)
- HIV
- TB

Do any of your family or friends have TB?

What is your occupation? (Assess for exposure to lung toxins—e.g., asbestos.)

How old are you?

What is the pattern of your sexual activity? (Assess for HIV risk.)

Do you smoke? How long, how much?

Differential diagnosis

Possible etiologies for abnormal CXR include:

- *Mycobacterium avium* complex
- HIV
- lymphoma
- lung primary
- metastatic cancer
- atypical pneumonia
- fungal pneumonia

Psychiatry and neurology

Case 77: Bipolar disorder

A 20-year-old man is experiencing severe mood swings. His concerned sister has accompanied him to his appointment. Please take a history and outline a management plan.

Time: 10 minutes

History

Some useful mnemonics for this history include:

- the **6Ss**: **s**leeping, **s**peaking, **s**pending, **s**ex, **s**elf-esteem, **s**uicide
- **AEA**: **a**ctivity, **e**nergy, **a**ppetite

The history needs to establish whether the symptoms last more than a week, and ask focused questions about depressive and manic symptoms. If a friend or family member accompanies the patient, get their perspective on the patient's symptoms (interview them with the patient or separately, as appropriate to the situation).

HISTORY OF PRESENT ILLNESS

When did your mood changes start?

What are they like?

How long do the moods last?

How are the moods affecting your life (e.g., school, work, home)?

How are your relationships with family and friends?

FOCUSED QUESTIONS: DEPRESSIVE SYMPTOMS

When your mood is down, how do the following aspects of your life change?

- sleep
- conversation
- libido
- self-esteem
- activities
- energy level
- appetite

Do you have suicidal thoughts?

FOCUSED QUESTIONS: MANIC SYMPTOMS

When your mood is up, do any of the following apply to you?

- sleeplessness
- flights of speech or ideas

How do the up moods affect the following?

- spending habits
- libido
- self-esteem
- activities
- energy levels
- appetite

PAST MEDICAL HISTORY

Have you had similar symptoms before? Have you been treated for them?

Have you ever attempted suicide?

Do any of the following apply to you?

- stroke
- trauma
- tumor
- infection
- endocrinopathy (hypo/hyperparathyroidism, Cushing disease, Addison disease, hypo/hyperthyroidism, insulinoma, pituitary disease)
- Parkinson disease

What medications do you take?

Do you have any family members with psychiatric disorders (e.g., mood disorder, schizophrenia, dementia)?

Who do you live with?

Do you have friends or family who help you?

What do you do for a living?

What do you do for recreation?

What do you typically eat for breakfast, lunch, and supper?

Do you drink alcohol? How much, how often?

Do you use recreational drugs?

Management

Certify and admit the patient if he is a risk to himself or others.

Rule out secondary causes such as other medical conditions (drug abuse, stroke, trauma, tumor, infection, endocrinopathy, Parkinson disease, nutritional deficiency) through a physical exam and blood work (urine drug screen, CBC, glucose, TSH, B_{12}).

Case 78: Anxiety

The wife of a 25-year-old man has brought her husband to you because he is experiencing anxiety. Please obtain a history.

Time: 5 minutes

History

The history needs to assess the severity of the condition, and its etiology as a psychiatric or other disorder.

HISTORY OF PRESENT ILLNESS

Is this an ongoing problem or a recent problem?

When did you begin experiencing the anxiety you are seeing me about today?

Are you aware of what may have triggered it (e.g., trauma, stress, drugs, exacerbation of another medical disorder)?

How long does the anxiety last?

Does anything make it better or worse?

How does the anxiety affect your usual activities (e.g., work, school, relationships)?

FOCUSED QUESTIONS: PSYCHIATRY ETIOLOGY

Do you experience any of the following?

- motor symptoms: tension, tremor, restlessness
- autonomic hyperactivity: shortness of breath, palpitations, sweating, cold clammy hands, dry mouth, dizziness, GI distress, excessive urination
- vigilance and scanning: exaggerated startle, concentration problems, sleep problems, irritability

Do you have any of the following symptoms (mnemonic: **STUDENTS fear 3Cs**)?

- **s**weating, **t**remor, **u**nsteadiness, **d**epersonalization, **e**xcessive heart rate, **n**ausea/vomiting, **t**ingling, **s**hortness of breath (STUDENTS)
- dying, loss of control, going crazy (fear)
- **c**hills, **c**hoking, **c**hest pain (3Cs)

Does anyone in your family have anxiety or other psychiatric conditions?

FOCUSED QUESTIONS: OTHER ETIOLOGY

Have you been diagnosed with any of the following?

- thyroid disease
- palpitations
- cardiac dysrhythmias
- pheochromocytoma
- Cushing syndrome
- hypoglycemia

What medications do you take (including prescription and over-the-counter medications)?

Do you drink alcohol? How much, how often?

Do you use recreational drugs?

Case 79: Schizophrenia

A 50-year-old woman, who had a hysterectomy 3 days ago, says she is hearing music and feels insects crawling on her. Please obtain a history and provide a mental disorder assessment.

Time: 10 minutes

History

Before you begin the history, assess whether the patient can give reliable information. If not, seek the information from another source (e.g., friend, family member).

HISTORY OF PRESENT ILLNESS

Is this an ongoing problem or a recent problem?

When did the current problem begin?

Do any of the following apply to you?

- feeling that people are against you
- hearing or seeing things that are not there, or that only you can appreciate (e.g., people talking to each other or talking to you)
- losing a sense of yourself or your environment (fugue state)
- believing others control your thoughts
- feeling you have a special mission

Do particular environments provoke symptoms?

How does the problem affect your usual activities (e.g., work, relationships)?

Do you have any of the following symptoms? (Assess for depression with mnemonic **SIG E CAPS**.)

- **s**leep changes
- **i**nterest changes (e.g., loss of interest)
- **g**uilt
- **e**nergy level changes
- **c**ognition/concentration changes
- **a**ppetite changes
- **p**sychomotor changes (agitation or retardation)
- **s**uicidal thoughts

Do you have thoughts of harming yourself or others?

Are you experiencing social or emotional stress in your life?

PAST MEDICAL HISTORY

Have you been diagnosed with a psychiatric disorder? Have you ever been treated or hospitalized for any psychiatric disorders?

Have you ever attempted suicide?

Have you been diagnosed with any chronic diseases?

What medications do you take?

Has anyone in your family experienced similar symptoms? Has anyone been diagnosed with a psychiatric disorder (e.g., depression, bipolar disorder)?

Do you have friends or family who help you?

How are your relationships with friends and family?

What was your situation growing up (e.g., complications before or during birth, or as an infant; family, school situation as a child or adolescent)?

Have you had any intimate partners as an adult? How have those relationships gone?

What is your occupation?

Do you drink alcohol? How much, how often?

Do you use recreational drugs?

Mental disorder assessment

Assessment should be based as much as possible on the *DSM-5* diagnostic categories:

- AXIS I Clinical disorder: consider mood disorder, schizophrenia, brief reactive psychosis, or other psychotic disorder
- AXIS II Personality disorder: difficult to assess in a limited interview situation
- AXIS III General medical condition (GMC): consider medication side effects, substance abuse, alcohol withdrawal
- AXIS IV Psychosocial and environmental: consider stressors
- AXIS V Global assessment of functioning (GAS): consider social/occupational dysfunction

Case 80: Somatization, conversion disorder

An elderly woman is experiencing multiple aches and pains. She has been seen by many physicians and has been extensively investigated with no diagnosis. She has seen your partner in your clinic and was not satisfied with their assessment, and so has come to you. Please take a history and discuss a management plan with the patient.

Time: 10 minutes

History

Because of the scenario, the history should focus on the possibility of somatization, with focused questions on primary and secondary gain.

During the history, stay alert to cues that the patient may have an organic disease.

HISTORY OF PRESENT ILLNESS

When did you start feeling this way?

Did the condition develop suddenly or gradually?

What are the symptoms like?

How frequent are they? How long do they last? Do they wake you up at night?

Does anything make the symptoms better or worse?

Are you experiencing any of the following?

- nausea, loss of appetite, vomiting, changes in bowel habits, weight changes (GI)
- shortness of breath, chest pain (cardiopulmonary)
- changes in libido, pain during sex (GU)
- changes in sensation, movement, or strength, or numbness or tingling (neurological)
- changes in interest levels, self-esteem, mood, ability to concentrate, activity or energy levels (depression)

What are your thoughts about your symptoms? Do you believe you have a serious illness? How do you cope?

PAST MEDICAL HISTORY

What medications do you take?

Do you have friends and family who help you?

Do you work? If so, what is your job?

How do the symptoms affect your daily life?

Have you been experiencing stress in your life (e.g., relationships, finances, work, stressful events)?

Are you worried about anything now?

FOCUSED QUESTIONS: SECONDARY GAIN

Who helps you when you are ill? What do they do?

What happens at work when you are ill?

Are you receiving disability payments?

Management

If you suspect an organic condition, recommend investigations as appropriate.

If you suspect somatization:

- Don't deny the patient's discomfort, or try to remove or cure symptoms: acknowledge the suffering and provide support.
- Avoid extensive further workup. Make the goal of care to help the patient adapt to chronic discomfort.
- Prescribe low dose medications (antidepressant, antianxiety, antipsychotic) as appropriate, but avoid extensive new medication.
- Address the patient's symptoms: research suggests that reassurance and education reduce anxiety. Assure the patient that the symptoms are self-limiting and should resolve.
- Manage the patient's internal conflict, as appropriate.
- Set up a schedule of appointments to further discuss issues and support the patient. Avoid "as needed" appointments.

Case 81: Anorexia nervosa

A mother brings her 16-year-old daughter to see you because she is concerned about her daughter's recent weight loss. You suspect anorexia nervosa. Please take a history, do a metal status exam (MSE), and discuss a management plan with the patient and her mother.

Time: 10 minutes

History

Note that you need to interview the patient separately from her mother.

HISTORY OF PRESENT ILLNESS

When did your eating habits change?

Have you been worrying about your weight? If so, for how long?

What do you think about your current weight?

How much do you think you should weigh?

Have you experienced weight changes recently? Over the last year, what has been your maximum and minimum weight?

How much do you weigh now? How tall are you? (Calculate body mass index.)

Do any of the following apply to you?

- fear of gaining weight
- preoccupation with diet and food
- depression (Assess with mnemonic **SIG E CAPS**: see Case 79.)
- skipped meals, diets, food binges, feeling fat
- induced vomiting (How often?)
- childhood abuse
- use of diet pills, laxatives, or diuretics for weight loss
- thoughts of suicide or self-harm

Do you have any of the following symptoms?

- feeling tired, dizzy, thirsty, cold
- hair or skin changes, abdominal pain
- rectal bleeding
- changes in menstrual periods

What do you typically eat for breakfast, lunch, and supper? What have you eaten in the last 24 hours?

What do you do for exercise (what type, how much)?

PAST MEDICAL HISTORY

Have you been diagnosed with any illnesses?

What medications do you take (prescribed and over-the-counter)?

How old were you when you had your first period? (Or—as appropriate—when your breasts began to develop?)

How long is your usual menstrual cycle? How many days of bleeding are usual for you? How many pads or tampons do you usually use per day?

Has there been any change in your cycle (timing, duration, quantity)?

Have you missed any periods?

Are you sexually active? What is the pattern of your sexual activity?

Who lives at home? How do you get along at home?

How are your usual activities going (e.g., school, job, recreation)?

How are your relationships with your friends?

Do you drink or use recreational drugs?

Mental status exam (MSE)

Assess:

- general appearance/behavior
- speech
- affect/mood
- thought process: circumstantial, tangential, flight of ideas, loosening of associations
- thought content: delusions (fixed false beliefs), obsessions, preoccupations
- dream content (recurrent themes), phobias, suicidal/homicidal ideation
- perceptions: hallucinations, illusions, depersonalization, derealization
- cognition: orientation, memory, intellectual functioning (concentration, abstract thought)
- judgment
- insight

Management

For anorexia nervosa, counsel the patient about:

- the importance of appropriate body weight for health
- symptoms related to weight loss: dizziness, cessation of periods, palpitations

- risks: serious arrhythmias and sudden death, irreversible erosion of tooth enamel, osteoporosis
- the need to resolve the mental and emotional sources of the problem

As appropriate:

- Refer the patient to a psychiatrist and specialized nutritionist.
- Refer the family to a family therapist.

Monitor the patient for weight, vitals, electrolytes, and cardiac complications (ECG).

Hospitalize the patient if the patient presents with:

- rapid, progressive weight loss
- persistent hypokalemia unresponsive to outpatient treatment
- less than 75% ideal body weight despite management
- bradycardia or hypotension
- refusal to eat

Consider the case urgent if the patient presents with:

- cardiac arrhythmias or severe bradycardia
- syncope
- dizziness
- severe depression or suicidality

Case 82: Depression

A young woman comes to you because she feels down. Please take a history, provide a differential diagnosis, and outline a management plan.

Time: 5 minutes

History

HISTORY OF PRESENT ILLNESS

When did you start feeling this way?

Is the feeling constant or intermittent?

Does anything make you feel better or worse?

Do any of the following apply to you? (Assess for organic etiology.)

- physical pain or discomfort
- symptoms of hypothyroidism (bradycardia, cold intolerance)
- past or current diagnosed illness
- past hospitalizations for illness or trauma

Do you have any of the following symptoms (mnemonic: **SIG E CAPS**)?

- **s**leep changes
- **i**nterest changes (e.g., loss of interest)
- **g**uilt
- **e**nergy level changes
- **c**ognition/concentration changes
- **a**ppetite changes
- **p**sychomotor changes (agitation or retardation)
- **s**uicidal thoughts

Do you have thoughts of harming others?

PAST MEDICAL HISTORY

Have you had similar episodes before?

Have you been treated before? If so, how did that go?

What medications are you taking?

Do you have any family members with similar problems?

What is your situation at home, work, and school?

Are you experiencing stress in your life (e.g., finances, friends, family)?

Who do you go to if you're in trouble?

Do you drink alcohol? How much, how often?

Do you use recreational drugs?

Differential diagnosis

Possible etiologies include:

- depression
- dysthymia
- bipolar disorder
- schizoaffective disorder
- hypothyroidism

Management

Treat any underlying medical conditions.

For psychological etiologies, as appropriate:

- Refer the patient for detox (substance abuse).
- Administer antidepressants.
- Refer the patient for psychotherapy.
- Hospitalize patients who have:
  - risk of homicide or suicide
  - inability to care for themselves
  - no family support
  - rapid progression of symptoms

Case 83: Suicide attempt

A 20-year-old man has attempted suicide by ingesting ASA. He is in hospital and medically cleared. Please do a psychiatric assessment.

Time: 5 minutes

History

Why did you try to kill yourself? Do you still want to kill yourself? Do you have a plan? Have you had other suicide attempts?

Do you know what may have triggered your suicide attempt (e.g., abuse, arguments, finances, school, peers, parents, siblings, work, loss of interest)?

Will the trigger still be there when you leave the hospital?

Do you have any past diagnosis of psychiatric illness or medical illness?

What medications do you take?

Do any of the following apply to you?

- hearing or seeing things that are not there; losing a sense of yourself or your environment; believing you are being controlled by outside influences
- recent mood changes
- panic or anxiety
- illness
- physical pain or discomfort
- changes in self-esteem

Do you have any of the following symptoms? (Assess for depression with mnemonic **SIG E CAPS.**)

- **s**leep changes
- **i**nterest changes (e.g., loss of interest)
- **g**uilt
- **e**nergy level changes
- **c**ognition/concentration changes
- **a**ppetite changes
- **p**sychomotor changes (agitation or retardation)
- **s**uicidal thoughts

Do you drink alcohol? How much, how often?

Do you use recreational drugs?

Do you abuse any over-the-counter medications?

What is your living situation (e.g., live alone, with family, with others)?

Do you have friends and family who help you?

Is there a history of suicide or similar situations in your family?

Psychiatric assessment

The psychiatric assessment includes an assessment of the patient's risk of succeeding in a suicide attempt and of the patient's family to respond if the patient needs help.

Keep in mind that certain patients have a higher risk of suicide (mnemonic: **SADPERSONS**):

- **s**ex: male
- **a**ge more than 60
- **d**epressed
- **p**revious attempts
- **e**thanol (alcohol) use

- **r**ationalized
- **s**uicide in family
- **o**rganized plan
- **n**o spouse
- **s**erious illness

PATIENT ASSESSMENT

The purpose of the patient assessment is to establish the intentions of the patient toward suicide (see breakdown that follows).

INTENTION	QUESTION TO PATIENT
Planned versus impulsive	Did you have a plan for killing yourself?
Lethality of attempt	How did you try to do it?
Chance of discovery	Where did you do it?
Reaction to being saved	How do you feel about being treated after your suicide attempt?
Triggers/causes/precipitants	Was there a specific event that led to your suicide attempt?
Prior attempts	Have you tried to kill yourself before?
Influence of drugs/alcohol	Were you drinking or on drugs when you tried to kill yourself?

FAMILY ASSESSMENT

The family assessment should include interviews with both the patient and members of the family. Assess whether the family can help the patient in terms of:

- appreciation of patient's condition/risk
- ability to handle crisis, provide support, monitor the patient
- access to other social supports
- history of psychiatric disorders

Management

Seek to make a contract with the patient: he should see you on a regular schedule, and contract to see you instead of harming himself.

Organize supports for the patient: refer him for counseling or to appropriate social agencies, depending on his needs.

Do not prescribe more than 1 week's supply (or total 1 g) of tricyclic antidepressants (TCAs) if there is a suicide risk.

Case 84: Suicide attempt by toxic ingestion

A patient is suspected of having taken an overdose of sleeping pills. Please initiate appropriate management.

Time: 5 minutes

Management

Suspect overdose when the following conditions apply:

- decreased LOC
- young patient with life-threatening arrhythmia
- trauma
- bizarre presentation

PRIMARY SURVEY

Ensure ABCs; provide oxygen; establish IV.

Initiate advanced cardiac life support (ACLS).

Administer a "coma cocktail":

- thiamine 100 mg IM/IV
- D50 glucose (50% in 100 mL)
- naloxone 2 mg IV, then 0.1 mg/kg (if suspect opioid overdose)

Initiate investigations:

- CBC, electrolytes, BUN, Cr, glucose, Mg, phosphate, Ca, LFTs
- ABG
- serum/urine osmolality
- drug tox screen
- ECG
- urinalysis

Decontaminate:

- ocular: irrigate
- skin: remove clothes
- GI: administer activated charcoal, gastric lavage, whole bowel irrigation
- GU: alkalinize urine
- assess for dialysis

Administer specific antidote if available.

Examine from head to toe.

Contact poison control center.

Case 85: Seizure

An 18-year-old patient presents with a seizure disorder and an increased number of seizures. Please take a history, do a physical exam, recommend investigations, and discuss a management plan with the patient.

Time: 10 minutes

History

The history needs to establish whether a true seizure has taken place. If possible, take information from the patient and from others who witnessed the seizure.

HISTORY OF PRESENT ILLNESS

How old were you when this problem began?

How often does it occur?

How long does an episode last?

Are any of the following associated with episodes?

- preceding aura
- eye movements
- vocalization
- loss of consciousness
- incontinence
- spread of symptoms from one body part to another

After an episode, do you feel confused or sleepy?

Have you noticed any triggers for episodes (e.g., sleep deprivation, alcohol, drugs)?

Do you have a fever or a rash?

PAST MEDICAL HISTORY

Have you had a previous diagnosis for this problem?

Have you had any treatment for this problem? If so, how did it affect the problem?

Are you taking any drugs for the problem?

- If so, what drugs and what doses?
- Do you sometimes miss doses?
  - If so, how frequently?
  - What happens?

What is the length of time between attacks?

Do any of the following apply to you?

- birth injury
- head trauma
- meningitis
- stroke
- developmental delay
- diabetes

Do you take benzodiazepine or insulin?

Has anyone in your family been diagnosed with seizures or other conditions?

Do you drink, smoke, or use recreational drugs?

Do live by yourself or with others?

Do you have a job? What do you do?

Physical exam

Check:

- ABCs
- vitals
- mental status

Perform:

- cranial nerves exam (see Table 23)
- cerebellar exam
- neurologic exam

Table 23. PROCEDURES FOR CRANIAL NERVES EXAM

CRANIAL NERVE	FUNCTION	SCREENING
I —sensory only	Olfaction	Assess ability to smell (test each nostril separately)
II —sensory only	Vision	Assess: • visual acuity (Snellen eye chart) • visual fields • pupillary light response Requisition: • fundoscopy
III —motor and sensory IV —motor only VI —motor only	III: EOM, pupillary constriction IV: Superior oblique muscle (SO4) VI: Lateral rectus muscle (LR6)	Assess: • eye movements • nystagmus • near reaction (accommodation) • pupillary constriction (III)
V —motor and sensory	Motor Sensory Reflexes (corneal and jaw-jerk)	Assess: • masseter and temporalis (muscles of mastication) • sensory: 3 distributions • reflexes
VII —motor and sensory	Motor Sensory anterior two-thirds of tongue	Assess: • ability to show teeth, squeeze eyes shut, puff out cheeks, raise eyebrows, whistle, tighten neck muscles • taste and sensation
VIII —sensory only	Hearing	Perform: • Webber test* • Rinne test** • otoscopy
IX —motor and sensory	Gag reflex Sensory posterior third of tongue	Assess: • gag reflex • taste and sensation

(Continued)

Table 23. (*Continued*)

CRANIAL NERVE	FUNCTION	SCREENING
X —motor and sensory	Palatal movement Gag reflex	Assess: • Ability to "say ahhh" • Ability to swallow • Uvula for deviation
XI —motor only	Sternomastoid Trapezius	Assess: • Ability to rotate head against resistance • Ability to shrug shoulders against resistance
XII —motor only	Tongue movement	Assess tongue for: • deviation (if nerve is damaged, tongue will deviate to the paralyzed side on protrusion) • atrophy/fasciculation

* Webber test: compares the ears for hearing acuity. The sound from a tuning fork placed in the center of the forehead should be the same in both ears. If there is a conductive hearing loss, the sound will lateralize to the "poor" ear.

** Rinne test: compares air conduction with bone conduction. With normal hearing, air conduction is greater than bone conduction. If there is a conductive hearing loss, bone conduction equals or is greater than air conduction.

Investigations

Recommend, as appropriate:

- EEG/imaging (CT or MRI of brain)
- CBC, electrolytes, Ca, phosphate, Mg, Cr
- random blood glucose
- liver enzymes
- lumbar puncture if you suspect infection
- anticonvulsant levels as needed

Management

Treat the underlying disease, as appropriate.

If the patient has a seizure disorder, educate the patient and family about the type of disorder (see Table 24 for an overview of seizure types).

Table 24. TYPES OF SEIZURES

CATEGORY	CHARACTERISTICS
Generalized	Involves loss of consciousness
	May involve: loss of bowel/bladder control, eyes rolling back (3–5 min), desaturation, postictal sleep
	Types:
	• tonic clonic: tonic phase where body becomes stiff with arms flexed (1–2 min) followed by clonic phase where repeated muscle spasms result in tongue biting
	• tonic
	• clonic
	• myoclonic
	• atonic
	• absence: patients are usually between preschool age and puberty, and experience shorter episodes of loss of consciousness
Partial (focal)	May involve an obvious organic etiology (e.g., tumor, scar) that causes aberrant electrical activity: the presentation can reflect the seizure focus
	Types:
	• simple partial: patients are still aware but experience motor, sensory, or autonomic changes
	• complex partial: patients experience disturbed consciousness, sometimes beginning as simple partial and then developing automatisms
Temporal lobe epilepsy	Begins with visual/olfactory sensation
Jacksonian march	Motor involvement starts with muscle groups at one location and progresses to involve muscle groups of adjoining motor cortex areas

Counsel the patient and family about:

- restricting or supervising activities such as swimming, boating, using heavy machinery, climbing heights, gum chewing, and using locked bathrooms
- pregnancy issues: close monitoring is required for female patients, some medications cause birth defects
- driving issues (licensing):
  - subject to local law
  - a seizure-free interval is required (usually 6 months to 1 year)
  - supervision by a physician is required
- support groups, which can be helpful

Schedule follow-up visits with the patient to ensure compliance and the efficacy of medications, and to monitor changes in symptoms.

Case 86: Neurological complications from alcoholism

A 35-year-old man with a history of alcoholism has just had a convulsion. Please perform a physical exam.

Time: 10 minutes

Physical exam

CATEGORY TO ASSESS	FINDINGS TO NOTE
Vitals	Hyperpyrexia, tachycardia
General appearance	LOC, nutritional status, diaphoresis
Head and neck	Angular cheilitis, parotitis, signs of liver disease
Abdomen	Signs of liver disease
Neurological status	
Mental status	Confusion, obtundation, dysarthria
	Depression
	Memory loss
	Hallucinations
Cranial nerves	Diplopia, nystagmus, cranial nerve VI palsy
Gait	Imbalance, ataxia

You can also assess the patient's neurological status by clinical presentation (see breakdown that follows).

CATEGORY	CLINICAL PRESENTATION
Acute intoxication	Slurred speech, CNS depression, disinhibited behavior, poor coordination
	Nystagmus, diplopia, dysarthria, ataxia (may progress to coma)
	Blackouts (possible subdural hematomas from falls)
Obtundation	Hypoglycemia
	Hepatic encephalopathy
Wernicke encephalopathy	Ocular nystagmus
	Sixth nerve palsy
	Gaze palsy
	Ataxia
	Vestibular dysfunction
	Vertigo, imbalance, delirium
Korsakoff syndrome	Marked short-term memory loss
	Difficulty learning new information (anterograde amnesia, confabulations)
Withdrawal	See Table 32

Case 87: Cerebellar dysfunction, ataxia

A 60-year-old man presents with difficulty walking. Please do a focused physical exam and provide a differential diagnosis.

Time: 5 minutes

Physical exam

Look for abnormalities in the rate, range, rhythm, and force of movement, without motor or sensory loss.

CATEGORY TO ASSESS	FINDINGS TO NOTE IF PRESENT
Vital signs	Hypotension
General appearance	Abnormal LOC, speech, affect
Gait and posture	Walking: abnormal initiation, stride length, arm movement; limping, tripping, more signs of wear on one shoe than the other
	Balance: staggering to one particular side, wide-based stance, en-bloc turning; loss of balance on Romberg test
	Decreased or asymmetric strength
Eyes	Nystagmus (fast component of beats favors the side of the lesion)
Speech	Dysarthria (scanning speech, staccato speech)
Unintentional movement	Dysdiadochokinesia (difficulty repeating alternating movements)
Intentional movement	Dysmetria (gross incoordination in finger-to-nose testing, heel-shin testing, and in rapid alternating movement)
	Intention tremor (e.g., when writing, pointing)
Motor	Impaired check/rebound and pendular reflex
	"Lead pipe" or "cogwheel" with resisted movement

Differential diagnosis

ETIOLOGY	SIGNS/SYMPTOMS
Nerve damage	Sensory loss and changes in reflex
	Symptoms that begin peripherally
	Abnormal nerve conduction studies
Muscle disease	Normal sensation and reflex
	Altered electromyography
Upper motor neuron lesion	Increased muscle tone, spasticity, hyperreflexia, Babinski sign
Lower motor neuron lesion	Flaccidity, hyporeflexia, fasciculations, atrophy

Case 88: Parkinson disease

A 60-year-old man presents with a tremor in his hands. Please take a focused history and do a focused physical exam to assess him for Parkinson disease.

Time: 5 minutes

History

HISTORY OF PRESENT ILLNESS

When did you first notice the tremor in your hands?

Is the tremor present at rest, when you hold your hands out, or when using your hands?

Is the tremor relieved by alcohol?

PAST MEDICAL HISTORY

Do you have a family history of tremor?

Physical exam

Look for (mnemonic: **TRAP**): **t**remor, **r**igidity, **a**kinesia, **p**ostural instability.

CATEGORY TO ASSESS	FINDINGS TO NOTE IF PRESENT
Vitals	Orthostatic change
General appearance	Masklike face, lack of blinking
	Blepharoclonus (fluttering of closed eyelids)
	Drooling: dysphagia and tongue protrusion
Speech	Dementia
	Hypophonia
Motor	Postural instability on standing
	Abnormalities in walking: starting hesitation, small shuffling steps, loss of arm swing, festination of gait, propulsion, stooped posture
	Abnormal arm movement: "cogwheel" rigidity, akinesia, bradykinesia
	Micrographia (small handwriting)
	Tremor: "pill rolling" tremor of the hand with a frequency of 4–7 times per second

Case 89: Meningitis

A teenage patient has had a recent URTI. For the last 2 days, the patient has been experiencing fever, vomiting, headache, and drowsiness. Please do a physical exam, provide a differential diagnosis, and recommend investigations.

Time: 10 minutes

Physical exam

CATEGORY TO ASSESS	FINDINGS TO NOTE IF PRESENT
ABCs	Signs of septic shock
Vitals	Any abnormal vitals, especially fever and hypotension
General appearance	Signs of toxic shock/sepsis
	Infectious focus (e.g., pneumonia, rash, heart murmur)
Neurologic status	Mental status: confusion
	Cranial nerves: pupils (nonresponsive to light/accommodation)
	Motor: paralysis, abnormal movement
	Pathological reflexes
	Altered sensation
	Head and neck: meningismus
	Reduced LOC (see Table 25)
	Meningeal irritation (see Table 26)

Table 25. GLASGOW COMA SCALE*

EYES	EXTREMITIES	SPEECH
1 Unresponsive: do not open	1 Do not respond (paralysis)	1 No speaking
2 Open in response to pain	2 Exhibit decerebrate response to pain (extension)	2 Makes incomprehensible sounds
3 Open in response to speech	3 Exhibit decorticate response to pain (abnormal flexing)	3 Says inappropriate words
4 Open spontaneously	3 Withdraw in response to pain	4 Makes confused conversation
	4 Demonstrate localized pain (patient can point to area)	5 Communicates well
	5 Respond to commands	

* Adapted from Teasdale G, Jennett B. Assessment of coma and impaired consciousness: a practical scale. *Lancet.* 1974;2(7872):81–84. doi:10.1016/S0140-6736(74)91639-0. PMID 4136544.

Interpretation: determine a score in each category and total the scores.

- total < 9: severely reduced LOC
- total 9–12: moderately reduced LOC
- total ≥ 13: mildly reduced LOC

Table 26. SIGNS OF MENINGEAL IRRITATION

SIGN	DETAILS
Nuchal rigidity	Patient experiences pain and resistance to passive neck flexion
Kernig sign	While supine and with hips flexed, patient experiences pain in the lower back and resistance to straightening the legs on extension
Brudzinski sign	When the neck is flexed, patient experiences involuntary flexion of hips and knees
Opisthotonus	Hyperextension of the back with arching

Differential diagnosis

Possible etiologies for this case include:

- meningitis
  - common causative agents of meningeal irritation (bacterial etiology):
    - infants: *E. coli*, *Listeria*, group B *Streptococcus*
    - 2–6 years: *H. influenzae*, *Streptococcus*
    - young: *N. meningitides*
    - 25 years and older: *S. pneumoniae*
- subarachnoid hemorrhage
- encephalitis
- trauma
- alcohol/drug intoxication

Investigations

If you suspect meningitis, recommend:

- CBC, electrolytes, blood and urine cultures, ESR, drug screen
- lumbar puncture: cerebrospinal fluid (CSF) opening pressures, cloudy, white blood count (neutrophils), protein (all increased but glucose low suggests bacterial cause)
- imaging: X-rays of chest/sinus/mastoid, CT, MRI
- EEG

Case 90: Coma

A comatose patient is brought to the emergency room. Please initiate appropriate management.

Time: 5 minutes

Management

PRIMARY SURVEY

Ensure ABCs. Check vitals including serum glucose.

Initiate resuscitation: start IV, oxygen; attach monitors.

Clear C-spine (lateral X-ray).

Initiate investigations:

- CBC, electrolytes, BUN, Cr, LFTs, serum osmolality, glucose
- ECG
- ABG
- urine drug screens

Give thiamine 100 mg IM before any glucose solutions:

- D5W: 50 mL if glucose is less than 4 or rapid measurement is not available
- naloxone 0.2–0.4 mg IV if narcotic toxidrome is present

Recheck vital signs.

SECONDARY SURVEY

Get a history from family, friends, witnesses, paramedics, police, etc. Ask about:

- onset: acute/gradual, preceding events
- trauma
- past medical history: diabetes, depression, cardiac disease, stroke/TIA, seizure
- medications
- use of alcohol, street drugs

Do a physical exam, with C-spine precautions (see breakdown that follows).

CATEGORY TO ASSESS	DETAILS
Vitals	BP, respiratory rate, temperature
Neurological status	Mental status (Glasgow coma scale: see Table 25)
	Cranial nerves:
	• pupils: symmetry, reaction to light
	• oculocephalic reflexes (**if** C-spine is cleared): normal = "doll's eyes"
	• oculocaloric reflexes (**first** R/O tympanic perforation): positive suggests dysfunction at lower brain stem
	Motor:
	• respiration rate and rhythm
	• apneic or ataxic (brain stem), Cheyne-Stokes respiration (cortical)
	• muscle tone, reflexes
Head and neck	"Raccoon" eyes, Battle sign
	Nuchal rigidity (**if** C-spine is cleared)
	Otorrhea, rhinorrhea, tongue biting, breath odor, hemotympanum/ perforation
	Jugular venous pressure:
	• depressed = dehydration, atrial fibrillation
	• bounding = tamponade, pulmonary embolus, right heart failure
Chest	Air entry, rales
Abdomen	Tenderness, guarding, signs of liver disease
Extremities	Needle track marks

TREATMENT

Definitive treatment depends on the specific cause and may involve consultation with ICU, neurology, or neurosurgery.

Establish supportive measures for the patient, as appropriate.

Case 91: Dementia

An elderly patient presents with decreased memory and increased confusion. Please take a history, perform a neurological exam, and outline a management plan.

Time: 10 minutes

History

The patient may not be able to provide reliable information, so aim to collect information from other sources as well, such as family and friends.

The history and the physical exam should both focus on distinguishing dementia from encephalopathy.

Keep in mind that depression often masquerades as dementia.

HISTORY OF PRESENT ILLNESS

When did this start?

Did it develop gradually or suddenly? (Assess dementia versus encephalopathy.)

Do you have any of the following symptoms?

- change in mood
- deterioration of memory
- difficulty finding the right words in conversation
- becoming lost while traveling along familiar routes
- difficulty with activities of daily living: dressing, cooking, washing, etc.

When the problem began to develop, what happened first? For example:

- loss in memory
- change in gait
- change in mood
- trauma (e.g., a fall)
- focal neurological signs (e.g., weakness in one side or part of the body, facial droop)

Is the problem getting better or worse?

How quickly is change happening?

Is change happening gradually or in steps? (Assess multi-infarct dementia versus diseases of neurodegeneration such as Alzheimer disease, endocrinopathy, Creutzfeldt-Jakob disease.)

Are you experiencing any of the following?

- loss of muscle coordination, urinary incontinence (normal pressure hydrocephalus)
- constipation, rough skin or hair, sluggishness, feeling cold (hypothyroidism)
- shuffling gait (Parkinson disease)
- step-wise progression, focal neurological signs (TIA/stroke)

PAST MEDICAL HISTORY

Have you been diagnosed with any of the following?

- high blood pressure or coronary artery disease
- diabetes
- transient ischemic attack (TIA) or stroke
- hypothyroidism
- anemia
- depression or other psychiatric issues
- chronic falls
- STDs

What medications do you take? For how long? Who are the prescribing physicians?

Are you taking your medications as prescribed?

Does your family have a history of dementia, depression, heart conditions, or stroke?

Are you living alone or with others?

Who helps you when you need help?

What do you usually eat for breakfast, lunch, and supper? Who prepares your meals?

Neurological exam

During the exam (see breakdown that follows), look specifically for:

- pseudodementia, depression, hypothyroidism
- degenerative processes, syphilis, anemia, B_{12} deficiency
- focality
- pseudobulbar signs (sudden cry/laugh with little provocation)

CATEGORY	DETAILS
Mental status	Formal testing: mini mental status exam (MMSE), frontal assessment battery testing, Montreal Cognitive Assessment (MoCA)
	Mood, affect, hallucination
Motor/cerebellar impairment	Involuntary movement
	Focal weakness or wasting
	Injuries
Reflexes	Primitive reflexes
Sensory impairment	Vision, hearing

Management

A multidisciplinary approach to management is ideal, using inputs from the fields of pharmacy, social work, physiotherapy, and occupational therapy. Consult a geriatrician as necessary.

Impaired function in the elderly tends to be multifactorial and some causes can be managed or treated to good effect (e.g., nutrition, reducing risk of falls).

Case 92: Dysphasia

A 58-year-old man presents with dysphasia. Please take a history and assess his status.

Time: 10 minutes

History

The patient may not be able to provide reliable information, so aim to collect information from other sources as well, such as family and friends.

HISTORY OF PRESENT ILLNESS

Which is your dominant hand?

What is your first language?

What level of education do you have?

Have you been diagnosed with a learning disability?

Assessment

The assessment should focus on:

- fluency
- paraphrasic errors (e.g., *dook* for *book*, *table* for *desk*)

- comprehension: verbal/written
- writing skills

ASSESSMENT INTERVIEW

Can you hear me?

Can you understand my questions?

Can you understand what people are talking about?

Can you repeat this phrase after me? (Say a phrase, such as "no ifs, ands, or buts.")

I'm going to point to some objects in the room. Can you tell me what they are?

What does this saying mean? "People who live in glass houses should not throw stones."

I'm going to write down something for you to do. Would you do it please? (Write down a command, such as "close your eyes.")

Would you please write down a complete sentence?

Case 93: Postoperative hallucination

A 50-year-old woman had a hysterectomy 4 days ago. She is now experiencing auditory and visual hallucinations. She was recently given Tylenol 3 and Ativan 1 mg. Please take a focused history and conduct an appropriate examination.

Time: 5 minutes

History

Do any of the following symptoms or factors apply to you? (See breakdown that follows.)

SYMPTOM/FACTOR	POSSIBLE ETIOLOGY
Heart palpitations, racing heart	Alcohol withdrawal/ delirium tremens
Shaking, tremors	
Agitation, anger	
Excessive sweating	
Alcohol abuse (How much? How often?)	
Epidural anesthesia during surgery (i.e., access to cerebrospinal fluid)	Encephalitis/meningitis
If yes:	
• discomfort at needle site	
• loss of consciousness	
• clinical signs of meningitis (see Table 26)	

(Continued)

SYMPTOM/FACTOR	POSSIBLE ETIOLOGY
Fever	Sepsis
Abnormal CBC/blood cultures	
Infection of wound	
Concurrent infections (e.g., pneumonia, UTI, cellulitis, abscess)	
Past similar episodes	Preexisting psychotic disorder
Seeing a doctor for psychiatric disorders (What doctors?)	
Taking medications for psychiatric disorders (Continuing or stopped?)	

Examination

Conduct a mini mental status exam, which evaluates a patient's sense of time and place (orientation); and ability to register information, perform mental tasks, recall information, and to use and process oral and written language. Please consult a textbook or online resource for details.

Case 94: Neurology assessment in neck injury

A patient has a neck injury. Please perform a neurological assessment.

Time: 5 minutes

Neurological exam

CATEGORY TO ASSESS	DETAILS
Motor responses	Muscle appearance, bulk, tone, power
	Deep tendon reflexes, abdominal and plantar responses
	Presence of involuntary movements (tics, tremors, myoclonus, chorea, hemiballismus, fasciculation)
Sensory responses	Response to pain, temperature, light touch
	Proprioception: Romberg test, joint position, 2 point discrimination
	Vibration sense
	Cortical sensory function, sensory suppression
	Reflexes
General neurological status	Vitals
	Lateralizing signs
	Cranial nerves: pupils
	Cerebellar function: Romberg test, gait, finger-to-nose test, heel-shin test, rapid alternating movement, nystagmus

Case 95: Stroke

A 60-year-old woman comes to the emergency room with new-onset left-sided hemiparesis and right-sided facial droop. Please take a history, perform a physical exam, provide a differential diagnosis, recommend investigations, and outline a management plan.

Time: 10 minutes

History

The patient may not be able to provide reliable information, so aim to collect information from other sources, such as the person who brought the patient to the emergency room.

HISTORY OF PRESENT ILLNESS

When did this happen?

Did anything trigger it (e.g., trauma)?

What were you (the patient) doing when this happened?

Did you have any of the following symptoms?

- loss of consciousness
- loss of bowel or bladder control
- seizure
- headache

Have you had any recent medical or dental procedures?

PAST MEDICAL HISTORY

Have you been diagnosed with any of the following?

- transient ischemic attack (TIA)
- atrial fibrillation
- high blood pressure
- coronary artery disease
- diabetes
- cancer
- hypercoagulability (blood clots)

What medications do you take?

Do any illnesses run in your family?

How old are you?

Do you smoke?

What do you do for a living?

Physical exam

Assess:

- ABCs
- mental status

Do a full neurological exam (sensory, motor, and cranial nerves) and a full cardiovascular exam (BP, heart sounds, carotid bruits, peripheral pulses).

Differential diagnosis

Possible etiologies for this case include:

- vascular abnormality (aneurysms, embolic phenomenon, ischemia, subarachnoid hemorrhage, intracranial hemorrhage)
- iatrogenesis
- trauma
- autoimmune abnormality (vasculitides)
- metabolic abnormality
- infection (meningitis, encephalitis)
- neoplasm
- congenital malformation
- degenerative disorder (dementias, neuromuscular, parkinsonism)

Investigations

Recommend:

- CT/MRI (ASAP)
- ECG
- CBC, electrolytes, BUN, Cr, glucose, PT, INR
- carotid Doppler, magnetic resonance (MR) angiography, echocardiogram

Management

Treat the underlying etiology.

If you suspect ischemic stroke:

- Administer thrombolytic, antiplatelet/ASA, anticoagulant, statin.
- Control risk factors such as DM, HTN, and smoking.

If you suspect hemorrhagic stroke:

- Avoid anticoagulants.
- Keep the patient inactive.

- Administer pain control.
- Refer for surgical decompression as necessary.

Case 96: Hearing loss

A 65-year-old man comes to your office with his wife. She says her husband is becoming hard of hearing. Please take a history, give a differential diagnosis, and recommend investigations.

Time: 5 minutes

History

The patient may not have the same perspective on his hearing as his wife. Take what they both say into consideration.

HISTORY OF PRESENT ILLNESS

When did you notice the loss of hearing?

How did you notice it?

Is the loss in one ear or both ears?

How has your hearing changed since you first noticed the loss (e.g., rapidly, slowly, no change)?

Do any of the following factors or conditions apply to you?

- ringing in the ears
- difficulties with balance
- ear pain
- recent ear infections
- recent other serious infection
- noise exposure

How do you remove your earwax?

PAST MEDICAL HISTORY

Have you ever had any of the following?

- vertigo
- head trauma
- stroke

What medications do you take (e.g., antibiotics, diuretics)?

Is there a history of hearing loss in your family?

What is your occupation? What occupations have you had in
the past?

What do you do for recreation or as a hobby?

Do you drink alcohol? How much, how often?

Differential diagnosis

See Table 27.

Table 27. DIFFERENTIAL DIAGNOSIS OF HEARING LOSS

CATEGORY	POSSIBLE ETIOLOGY
Conductive	Tympanic membrane perforation
	Cerumen impaction
	Foreign body
Sensory	Aging: senile presbycusis
	Infection
	Noise exposure
	Toxic medication
Neural	Infection
	Trauma
	Stroke
	Tumor

Investigations

Recommend audiometry.

Case 97: Sleep disorder

A 40-year-old woman says she is having difficulty sleeping. Please take a history, do a physical exam, recommend investigations, and discuss a management plan with the patient.

Time: 5 minutes

History

If the patient has a spouse or partner, collect information from that person, too.

HISTORY OF PRESENT ILLNESS

When did you start having difficulty sleeping?

Is the problem constant or intermittent? If intermittent, how long do episodes last?

What part of sleep do you have difficulty with (e.g., falling asleep, frequent waking, early waking)?

What is your sleep environment like for noise, temperature, and light?

What do you do when you are unable to sleep? (Assess whether the patient is engaging in stimulating activities, such as watching TV or checking e-mail.)

Do any of the following apply to you?

- shift work
- alcohol use
- recreational drug use
- smoking
- stress
- morning headaches
- manic symptoms

Do you have any of the following during sleep? (Check with the patient's partner, if possible.)

- cessation of breathing (sleep apnea)
- restless legs
- snoring

How does the problem affect your daily activities (e.g., work, recreation)?

PAST MEDICAL HISTORY

Have you been diagnosed with any of the following?

- hyperthyroidism
- frequent upper respiratory tract infections
- allergies

What medications do you take?

Does anyone in your family snore?

Physical exam

Look for signs of sleep apnea (obesity, micrognathia, HTN, etc.) and thyroid disease.

Examine the oral cavity and neck for masses.

Investigations

Recommend:

- a sleep diary kept by the patient (patient records bedtime, time to falling asleep, nighttime waking, time of waking, and sleep quality)
- CBC, TSH
- referral for sleep studies, as appropriate

Management

Treat any specific medical or psychiatric cause.

Counsel the patient about:

- snoring and obstructive sleep apnea, as appropriate (see Table 28 and Table 29)
- sleep hygiene: avoid caffeine, use bed for sleep and sex only, exercise regularly, keep a regular sleep schedule
- relaxation therapy and counseling if indicated
- sleep restriction: limit time in bed to time required for sleeping

Prescribe short-term benzodiazepine therapy (especially if the patient has a specific transient cause for inability to sleep).

Table 28. SNORING: RISK FACTORS AND TREATMENT

RISK FACTORS	TREATMENT
Male > female	Sleep on side
Obesity	Lose weight
Alcohol use	Use nasal dilators
Tranquilizer use	Use alcohol, tranquilizers in moderation
Smoking	Stop smoking
Nasal polyps	

Table 29. OBSTRUCTIVE SLEEP APNEA: RISK FACTORS, CONSEQUENCES, AND TREATMENT

RISK FACTORS	CONSEQUENCES	TREATMENT
Obesity	Daytime sleepiness	No supine sleeping
Tonsils or adenoids in children	Nonrestorative sleep	Weight loss
Aging	Interference with work performance	Avoidance of triggers for poor sleep (e.g., alcohol)
Persistent URTIs	Mood changes	Continuous positive airway pressure (CPAP) machine
Allergies	Sexual dysfunction	
Nasal tumors	Morning headache (hypercapnia)	
Hypothyroidism (macroglossia)	HTN	Surgery: not effective in cases caused by obesity but may be helpful in children
Family history of snoring	Coronary artery disease	
	Stroke	
	Arrhythmias	
	Decreased concentration	

Case 98: Smoking cessation

A 50-year-old man who is a heavy smoker has come to you for advice on how to quit smoking. Please discuss a management plan with the patient.

Time: 10 minutes

Management

Offer treatment to every smoking patient (mnemonic: **5As**):

- **a**sk about smoking
- **a**dvise to quit
- **a**ssess stage of change/willingness to quit (see Table 30)
- **a**ssist in quitting
- **a**rrange follow-up

Table 30. STAGES OF CHANGE IN BEHAVIOR MODIFICATION*

STAGE	DETAILS
Precontemplation	Patient: denies/ignores information about the consequences of behavior (e.g., smoking)
	Physician's role: encourage the patient to change and assess patient's readiness to change
Contemplation	Patient: feels ambivalent about change
	Physician's role: encourage change and discuss benefits of change with patient
Preparation	Patient: wants to discuss options and address concerns
	Physician's role: respond
Action	Patient: undertakes change
	Physician's role: provide positive reinforcement, address patient's obstacles to change
Maintenance	Patient: seeks to maintain change
	Physician's role: maintain motivation and try to prevent relapse
Relapse	Patient: feels discouraged about relapse
	Physician's role: be nonjudgmental, help patient to understand reasons for relapse, and begin the process again

* Adapted from Prochaska JO, DiClemente CC. Stages and processes of self-change of smoking: toward an integrative model of change. *J Consult Clin Psychol.* 1983;51(3):390–395.

Discuss the patient's smoking habits, previous attempts to quit, and results of attempts to quit.

Schedule 4 or more counseling sessions of at least 10 minutes for the next 6 to 12 months. The highest risk of relapse in a recent quitter is in the first

3 months. Assist these patients by providing positive reinforcement, by anticipating challenges, and with frequent follow up.

Address the patient's concerns with quitting (e.g., weight gain).

Reinforce the benefits of quitting (e.g., financial gain, physical appearance).

Provide access to community support and behavioral modification.

Recommend nicotine replacement therapies: gum, patch, inhaler, nasal spray.

Prescribe medications, as necessary (e.g., bupropion, Champix).

Case 99: Alcoholism

An alcoholic has been charged with drunk driving and wants help to stop drinking. Please take a history and discuss a management plan with the patient.

Time: 10 minutes

History

HISTORY OF PRESENT ILLNESS

What are your drinking habits?

- frequency
- quantity consumed in a week
- when: times in the day, days of the week, occasions
- where
- alone or with others

Do you want to drink, or do you have to drink?

How has drinking affected your home life, work life, and relationships?

Do you have any safety concerns when you drink (e.g., accidents, arrests, drinking and driving, suicidal thoughts)?

Why do you drink? (Assess for mood, coping mechanism.)

How do you feel about your drinking? (Assess for alcoholism with mnemonic **CAGE**: **c**ut down, **a**nnoyed, **g**uilty, **e**ye opener.)

- Have you ever wanted to cut down?
- Have people annoyed you by criticizing your drinking?
- Have you ever felt guilty about drinking?
- Do you feel you need an "eye opener" in the morning?

PAST MEDICAL HISTORY

Have you been diagnosed with any illnesses?

What medications are you taking?

Do you use recreational drugs?

What is your occupation?

What are your living arrangements?

Management

Assess the patient's stage of change (see Table 30) and provide counseling as appropriate.

Discuss with the patient the medical problems related to alcoholism (see Table 31) and review the detrimental effects of alcoholism on relationships, work, etc.

Table 31. MEDICAL PROBLEMS RELATED TO ALCOHOLISM

CATEGORY	SEQUELAE
GI	Bleeds, liver disease, pancreatitis, oroesophageal cancer
Heart	Cardiomyopathy
Lung	Aspiration
Neurologic system	Double vision, nystagmus, gait abnormalities, forgetfulness, confabulation (Wernicke/Korsakoff encephalopathy)
Hematological system	Anemia, coagulopathy

Address the patient's fears and concerns about treatment, for example:

- symptoms of withdrawal (see Table 32)
- underlying reasons for drinking

Table 32. SYMPTOMS OF WITHDRAWAL FROM ALCOHOL ADDICTION

TIMING, POST DRINKING*	SYMPTOMS
6–8 hours	Generalized anxiety, agitation, tremor, insomnia, nausea/vomiting
24–36 hours	Visual/auditory hallucinations
24–48 hours+	Seizures (generalized tonic-clonic)
	Delirium tremens: severe confusion, hyperpyrexia, diaphoresis, agitation, insomnia, hallucination/delusion, tremor, tachycardia

* timing of symptoms may vary widely among individuals

Discuss options for social and community support (e.g., Alcoholics Anonymous). Refer the patient for psychiatric or behavior-modification intervention, as appropriate. Encourage self-monitoring.

Involve family or significant others in treatment, and get treatment for them as well.

Make a schedule of regular follow-up appointments with the patient.

Prescribe drugs as appropriate:

- for dependence and abuse: disulfiram
- for withdrawal: benzodiazepines, beta-blockers, thiamine

Case 100: Lump in throat

A 55-year-old woman says she feels a lump in her throat when she swallows. Please take a focused history.

Time: 5 minutes

History

HISTORY OF PRESENT ILLNESS

When did you first notice this problem?

Has it changed since you noticed it?

Is the problem constant or intermittent?

Do you have difficulty swallowing? If yes, has there been a progression in difficulty (e.g., from just solids to solids and liquids)?

Do you have any of the following symptoms?

- pain with swallowing
- night sweats, weight loss
- heartburn, indigestion, acid taste in mouth

Have you had any recent infections?

Have you had any recent stress in your life?

PAST MEDICAL HISTORY

Have you been diagnosed with any illnesses (e.g., thyroid problems, GI reflux, cancer)?

What medications do you take?

Do any diseases run in your family?

What do you do for a living?

Do you drink or smoke?

Case 101: Visual disturbances

A 70-year-old man is experiencing visual disturbances. Please take a focused history.

Time: 5 minutes

History

The history should aim to rule out temporal arteritis and central retinal artery occlusion, both of which require emergency treatment.

HISTORY OF PRESENT ILLNESS

When did the visual disturbance start?

Did it develop suddenly or gradually?

What is the problem (e.g., loss of vision, seeing double)?

If vision loss:

- Is the problem in one eye or both eyes?
- Is it confined to one area of the visual field?

If diplopia:

- Is it relieved by covering one eye?
- Is the double image horizontal, vertical, or oblique?
- Is it worse in one direction of gaze?
- Is it fluctuating or constant?

Do you have a change in color perception?

Do any of the following apply to you?

- history of trauma, headache
- fatigue, joint symptoms, weight loss, night sweats, fever
- severe headaches, jaw pain

PAST MEDICAL HISTORY

Have you been diagnosed with any illnesses?

What medications do you take?

Does anyone in your family have similar symptoms?

Do any diseases run in your family?

How old are you?

What is or was your occupation?

Do you drink or use recreational drugs?

Do you have a history of smoking?

Case 102: Hoarseness

A 55-year-old man has a hoarse voice. Please take a history, provide a differential diagnosis, and recommend investigations.

Time: 5 minutes

History

As you take the history, note the patient's character of voice, which can relate to etiology:

- breathy: cord apposition due to tumor, polyp, nodule
- raspy: cord thickening, edema, or inflammation due to infection, chemical irritation, or voice abuse
- high/shaking or soft: trouble mounting adequate respiratory force

HISTORY OF PRESENT ILLNESS

When did the hoarseness begin?

Did it develop suddenly or gradually?

Does anything make it better or worse?

Is it generally getting better or worse?

Do any of the following apply to you?

- abuse of voice (e.g., singing, speaking for theatre, crying, shouting)
- fever, sore throat, muscle aches/pains (Assess for recent URTI.)
- throat pain at rest, with voice use, with swallowing
- difficulty breathing, swallowing, talking (Note: stridor or difficulty breathing is an emergency!)
- worse with talking
- weight loss, neck mass, chest pain, coughing, blood in what you cough up

Do you have any psychological concerns?

PAST MEDICAL HISTORY

Have you had any recent medical procedures (e.g., endoscopy, tubes down throat, anesthesia, thyroid surgery)?

Have you been diagnosed with thyroid disease?

Do you have any allergies?

What medications do you take?

Do any diseases run in your family (e.g., thyroid disease, environmental allergies)?

How old are you?

What is your occupation? What do you do for recreation? (Assess for exposure to dust and fumes.)

Do you drink or smoke?

Differential diagnosis

Acute etiologies for hoarseness include:

- laryngitis: viral infection, vocal abuse, toxic fumes, allergy
- laryngeal edema: angioneurotic, infection, direct injury, nephritis, epiglottitis

Chronic etiologies include:

- laryngitis: vocal abuse, smoking, allergy, persistent irritant exposure
- laryngeal lesions: polyps, leukoplakia, contact ulcer, granuloma, nodules, benign/malignant tumor
- vocal paralysis: brain stem lesion, laryngeal nerve injury, aortic aneurysm, tumor, surgery
- vocal cord trauma: chronic intubation
- systemic abnormalities: hypothyroidism, rheumatoid arthritis (RA), virilization
- psychogenic conditions

Investigations

Hoarseness for more than 2 to 3 weeks requires an exam of the larynx to rule out malignancy. Recommend, as appropriate:

- laryngoscopy
- biopsy of any observed lesions
- CT/MRI of neck
- CRP, TSH

Case 103: Dizziness, vertigo

A 35-year-old man presents with dizziness. Please take a focused history, do a physical exam, provide a differential diagnosis, and recommend investigations.

Time: 10 minutes

History

The history needs to establish if the patient is experiencing vertigo and focus on etiology.

HISTORY OF PRESENT ILLNESS

When did the problem begin?

Did it develop suddenly or gradually?

Is it constant or intermittent?

What characterizes the dizziness?

- sensation of rotation
- lightheadedness
- confusion
- feeling giddy or dazed

Is the dizziness accompanied by an unsteady gait?

Is it triggered by certain movements, head positions, standing, or turning?

Does it get worse with eyes closed or with movement?

How long does it last (e.g., seconds, minutes, hours, days, months)?

What other symptoms do you have with the dizziness (e.g., blurry vision, loss of coordination, ear/hearing symptoms, nausea or vomiting)?

PAST MEDICAL HISTORY

Have you been treated for this problem before? With what results?

Have you been diagnosed with any of the following?

- Ménière disease
- stroke
- diabetes
- chronic obstructive pulmonary disease
- heart disease
- depression

What medications do you take? Have you taken gentamicin recently?

Does anyone in your family have similar symptoms?

Do any diseases run in your family?

How old are you?

What do you do for a living?

Physical exam

Check:

- eyes: nystagmus, fundoscopy
- cranial nerves: especially CN V (see Table 23)
- ears: otoscopy, tuning fork tests

Also check for:

- long-tract signs: cerebellar, pyramidal, sensory
- benign paroxysmal positional vertigo (BPPV): Dix-Hallpike test

Differential diagnosis

ETIOLOGY	SIGNS/SYMPTOMS
Vertigo	
Central: brain stem, cerebellar caused by tumor, stroke, drugs	Sensation of rotation, worse with eyes closed or with movement
	Duration: days (acute)
	Diplopia, dysphasia, ataxia
Peripheral: inner ear, vestibular nerve, Ménière disease, benign paroxysmal positional vertigo (BPPV)	Sensation of rotation, worse with eyes closed or with movement
	Duration: minutes to 24 h (Ménière disease), days (acute)
	Hearing loss, tinnitus, otalgia, labyrinthitis, pressure in the ear
Nonvertigo	
Ocular	Decreased visual acuity
Vascular: vertebrobasilar insufficiency, TIA, basilar migraine, orthostatic hypotension, arrhythmia, CHF, aortic stenosis, stroke	Sensation on changing position (supine to standing)
	Duration: a minute
Metabolic: hypoxia, hypoglycemia, hyper/hypocapnia	Low PO_2, abnormal PCO_2, low blood glucose

(Continued)

ETIOLOGY	SIGNS/SYMPTOMS
Psychiatric: anxiety, depression, psychosis	Symptoms of depression (mnemonic **SIG E CAPS**):
	• **s**leep changes
	• **i**nterest changes (e.g., loss of interest)
	• **g**uilt
	• **e**nergy level changes
	• **c**ognition/concentration changes
	• **a**ppetite changes
	• **p**sychomotor changes (agitation or retardation)
	• **s**uicidal thoughts

Investigations

Recommend:

- audiometry, caloric testing
- evoked potentials, CT/MRI

Case 104: Headache

A patient presents with a history of headache. Please obtain a history, perform a physical exam, provide a differential diagnosis, recommend investigations, and outline a management plan.

Time: 10 minutes

History

Be aware of emergency warning signs, such as new onset, sudden onset, "worst headache ever," associated fever, projectile vomiting, deteriorating LOC, focal neurological signs, head injury, and optic disc edema.

HISTORY OF PRESENT ILLNESS

Is this a new headache, or have you had similar headaches in the past?
If new headache:

- When did it start?
- Did it develop suddenly or gradually?
- Do you know what triggered it (e.g., trauma)?

- Is it constant or intermittent? If intermittent, how frequently does the pain occur? How long does it last?

If chronic headache:

- Have you experienced a change in headaches?
- How old were you when the headaches began?
- Is there any pattern of occurrence (e.g., same time of day, sudden/gradual development)?
- Do you know of any triggers (e.g., fever, fatigue, stress, food, alcohol, allergy, menstrual cycle)?
- How long do the headaches last (minutes, hours, days, weeks)? Are there any pain-free periods?
- How frequent are the headaches?
- Do the headaches occur in clusters?
- What is a typical episode like (before, during, after)?
- Are the headaches preceded by symptoms (e.g., aura)?

Where is the pain (e.g., entire head, unilateral, specific site)?

- Chronic headache: always in the same spot?

What is the pain like (e.g., throbbing, pounding, constant pressure, tightening band, piercing)?

Does the pain radiate to other parts of your head or body?

How severe is the pain on a scale of 1 (low) to 10 (high)?

Is the pain worse in the morning, as the day progresses, or during the night?

Does anything make the pain worse (e.g., movement, light, sound)?

Does anything make it better (e.g., medication, sleep, other treatment)?

Do you have any of the following symptoms?

- nausea, vomiting, fever, loss of consciousness, altered sensation in extremities, change in strength
- problems with vision, hearing, smell, bite
- nasal or ear discharge
- watery eyes, light sensitivity, neck stiffness, seizures
- pain in the jaw or ear while chewing

PAST MEDICAL HISTORY

Do any of the following apply to you?

- head trauma
- recent lumbar puncture

- surgery
- seizure

What medications do you take?

Does anyone in your family experience headaches similar to yours?

Does your family have a history of thyroid dysfunction, brain tumor, cancers, or other medical problems?

What is your occupation? What do you do for recreation? (Assess for risk of head injury, exposure to toxins.)

Are you experiencing stress in your life (e.g., home, work, school)?

What do you usually eat for breakfast, lunch, and dinner? Do you skip meals? Have your eating habits changed (e.g., for dieting)? (Assess nutritional status.)

Do you drink, smoke, or use recreational drugs?

Physical exam

CATEGORY TO ASSESS	FINDINGS TO NOTE, IF PRESENT
Vitals	Abnormalities in BP, pulse, respiration rate, temperature
Head	Abnormalities in general appearance (skin, hair, scars, location of pain)
	Arteries: carotid, temporal, occipital (bruits, tender, pulsating)
	Temporomandibular joint (tenderness, crepitus, locking)
Nose	Discharge, sinus tenderness, translucence
Ear	Discharge, hearing, mastoid
Eyes	Corneal clouding (glaucoma)
	Abnormalities in pupils, vision, fundoscopy, intraocular pressure
Oral cavity	Teeth, trigger points for pain
Cranial nerves	Motor or sensory deficits
C-spine	Rigidity, tenderness
Neurological system	Ataxia, LOC, focal neurological deficits

Differential diagnosis

Headaches can have an intracranial or extracranial source (see breakdown that follows).

INTRACRANIAL	EXTRACRANIAL
Mass, cerebrovascular, migraine, meningitis, postconcussion	Tension, sinusitis, temporal arteritis, temporomandibular joint, cluster, indomethacin responsive, systemic infection/fever, HTN, ocular, cervical radiculopathy, trigeminal neuralgia

Possible etiologies of chronic recurrent headache include:

- muscle contraction: tension headache, psychogenic, depression, anxiety, stress
- cervical osteoarthritis
- temporomandibular joint (TMJ) disease
- vascular abnormalities
- migraine
- cluster headache
- drugs (e.g., overuse of analgesics)

Possible etiologies of acute headache include:

- infection: meningitis, encephalitis
- posttrauma conditions: concussion, cerebral contusion, subdural/epidural hematoma
- vascular abnormalities: subarachnoid hemorrhage, intracerebral hemorrhage
- elevated intracranial pressure: space-occupying lesion, malignant HTN, benign intracranial HTN
- temporal arteritis, acute angle closure glaucoma

Investigations

Recommend, as appropriate:

- CBC, ESR, cerebrospinal fluid (CSF)
- plain sinus X-rays, CT, MRI, arteriography
- other: temporal artery biopsy, spinal tap (rule out infection/bleed)

Management

The breakdown that follows describes management for common conditions causing headache.

ETIOLOGY	TREATMENT
Migraine	Prevention: avoidance of triggers; NSAIDs, physiotherapy, calcium channel blocker (verapamil), triptans, topiramate
	Treatment of aura: aspirin, ergotamine
	Treatment of full-blown headache: ergotamine, meperidine, antiemetic, fluid hydration
Tension headache	Acetaminophen, NSAIDs, physiotherapy, antidepressants

(*Continued*)

ETIOLOGY	TREATMENT
Cluster headache	Avoidance of alcohol
	Oxygen, ergotamine, NSAIDs, verapamil, prednisone
Temporal arteritis	Administer prednisone 60 mg orally immediately to prevent blindness; maintain dose until symptoms resolve, then taper
Concussion	Rest until symptom free, then supervised gradual increase in activities
Medication overuse headache	Discontinuation of overused medication and initiation of prophylactic medication

Case 105: Drug seeker

A 20-year-old man from out of town wants Fiorinal for headaches. Please take a history and discuss a management plan with the patient.

Time: 5 minutes

History

The history needs to establish whether the patient is abusing the drug he is seeking.

HISTORY OF PRESENT ILLNESS

Do you have a headache now?

What is the frequency and severity of your headaches?

What is a typical headache like (timing, duration, triggers, pain quality)?

Does anything make the pain better or worse?

What symptoms are associated with your headaches (e.g., nausea, vomiting, vision changes, auras)?

Have you had the headaches investigated for cause?

When was your last prescription for Fiorinal?

Who prescribes for you normally?

Do you have your bottle with you?

Management

Attempt to reach the patient's primary physician. With the permission of the primary physician, consider prescribing a very limited supply of Fiorinal (several pills only).

If the patient does not have a "narcotics contract," ask him to form one with his primary physician. This contract is an agreement that the patient will only get prescriptions from one physician, will not receive early refills, will not sell the prescribed drug, or use it for any purpose other than the prescribed reason.

If you suspect the patient is abusing Fiorinal (e.g., the patient's bottle shows a recent prescription and a large dose gone):

- Do not prescribe Fiorinal.
- Educate the patient about Fiorinal: it is a combination analgesic and sedative consisting of acetaminophen or aspirin, butalbital, and caffeine. Taking Fiorinal can give a high with increased energy and confidence, and may be addictive. Frequent use in high doses can cause tachycardia, fever, interstitial nephritis, etc.
- Recommend the patient establish an effective headache-prevention regimen, to avoid regular use of Fiorinal.
- Offer alternative treatments for headache until the patient can return to his regular prescriber.

Surgery

Case 106: Nipple discharge

A 60-year-old woman presents with nipple discharge. Her mammogram shows microcalcification. Please take a history and discuss a management plan with the patient.

Time: 5 minutes

History

HISTORY OF PRESENT ILLNESS

When did you first notice the discharge?

What color is it (e.g., bloody, yellow, green, white)? How much is there? Does it have an odor?

Is the discharge from one breast or both breasts?

Does it seem to come from one spot or multiple spots in the nipple?

Is it spontaneous, intermittent, or persistent? Is it produced by pressure at a specific spot or all over?

Is the discharge painful?

Is there any change in the skin of the breast? Have you felt a mass in the breast or the areas around the breast (axilla)?

Are you otherwise healthy? Have you experienced fever, cough, bone pain, or weight loss?

PAST MEDICAL HISTORY

Have you ever had breast cancer or other breast diseases (e.g., cysts, fibrocystic disease)?

What medications are you taking (e.g., hormone replacement therapy)?

Has anyone in your family had breast cancer?

Are you still menstruating? Have you had any change in your menstrual periods?

How old were you when you had your first period?

If menopausal, how old were you when you stopped menstruating?

Have you ever been pregnant? If so, how many times?

How many children do you have?

Did you breast-feed? Did you have any difficulties breast-feeding?

Do you smoke, drink, or take recreational drugs?

Management

Counsel the patient that:

- Nipple discharge can be associated with fibrocystic change, intraductal papilloma, or hormonal influences.
- Microcalcifications can be associated with benign breast disease such as fibrocystic change, or with cancers such as ductal carcinoma in situ and invasive carcinoma.
- A core biopsy of the calcification area is essential to rule out cancer.
- If the nipple discharge is bloody, needle-localized excisional biopsy can have both diagnostic and therapeutic value.
- Further investigations for metastasis include: CXR, bone scan, etc.
- Prognosis is determined by size, stage, local invasion, lymph node status, distant metastases, estrogen receptor status, etc.

Case 107: Carpal tunnel syndrome

A patient presents with wrist pain and finger numbness. Please take a history, do a focused physical exam, provide a differential diagnosis, recommend investigations, and outline a management strategy.

Time: 10 minutes

History

Be alert for risk factors: occupational (repeated mild movements/trauma), pregnancy, acromegaly, myxedema, diabetes, and inflammatory arthritis.

HISTORY OF PRESENT ILLNESS

When did the problem begin?

Did it begin suddenly or gradually?

On a scale of 1 (low) to 10 (high), how bad is your pain?

How does this pain affect your daily life?

Does anything make the pain better or worse (e.g., certain activities)?

Do you have any of the following symptoms?

- numbness in your hands or fingers
- joint pain other than in your wrist and hands
- fever, weight loss, fatigue, night sweats

PAST MEDICAL HISTORY

Have you ever had surgery or trauma to your wrists or hands?

Is there a history of arthritis in your family?

What is your occupation?

What do you do for recreation?

Physical exam

Always examine the joints above and below any affected joint.

CATEGORY TO ASSESS	DETAILS
Neck, shoulder, elbows, arm	Palpation: pain, tenderness, point tenderness in specific parts of neck or shoulder
Forearm and wrist	Inspection: size of forearm, compare both sides, deformity
	Palpation: tender points, anatomical snuffbox, crepitus
	ROM: flexion-extension, radial-ulnar deviation

(Continued)

CATEGORY TO ASSESS	DETAILS
Forearm and wrist (continued)	Muscles: flexors (flexor carpi radialis/ulnaris, flexor digitorum sublimis/profundus), extensors (extensor carpi radialis longus/ulnaris, extensor digitorum, extensor pollicis longus)
Hand	Inspection: deformity, skin, nails, tendon thickening, muscle wasting, fasciculations
	Palpation: every bone and joint (swelling, tenderness, Heberden nodule at distal interphalangeal joint, Bouchard nodule at proximal interphalangeal joint)
	ROM: finger (flexion-extension, adduction-abduction) thumb (flexion-extension, adduction-opposition)
Nerves	Ulnar nerve (first digital interosseus, adductor pollicis, abductor digital minimi)
	Median nerve (thenar eminence, abductor pollicis brevis, opponens pollicis)

Differential diagnosis

Positive signs of carpal tunnel syndrome include:

- numbness: thumb, index and long fingers, radial side of ring finger
- thenar atrophy and finger weakness
- Phelan test: symptoms reproduced with 1 minute of palmar flexion
- Tinel test: symptoms reproduced with tapping on the median nerve

Other etiologies for wrist pain and finger numbness include:

- C-spine source, thoracic outlet syndrome
- nerve entrapment syndrome
- arthritis
- tendonitis

Investigations

As appropriate, recommend:

- nerve conduction studies (nerve conduction velocity)
- electromyography (EMG)
- X-rays: C-spine, wrist, hand

Management

Recommend, as appropriate:

- weight loss, furosemide
- rest and nighttime splinting

- NSAIDs
- steroid injections

Surgical release is indicated for:

- refractory pain (more than 3 months)
- sensory loss
- muscle atrophy

Case 108: Abdominal pain

A patient presents with acute abdominal pain. Please do a physical exam, provide a differential diagnosis, and recommend investigations.

Time: 10 minutes

History

HISTORY OF PRESENT ILLNESS

When did the pain start?

Did it develop suddenly or gradually?

Does the pain radiate to other parts of your body?

Where is the pain (e.g., generalized or localized)?

At which spot does it hurt the most?

Is the pain associated with bowel movements? Have you had changes in bowel habits?

Is the pain constant or intermittent (colicky)?

Do you have pain at night? Does it wake you up?

Does the pain have association with meals, breathing, certain foods?

Do you have any of the following symptoms?

- nausea, vomiting (Check quality of vomitus: bloody, bilious, undigested food.)
- diarrhea
- constipation
- gas
- passing nothing by rectum
- change in appetite or weight
- fever, chills, sweats
- urinary changes (e.g., pain)

Are you experiencing stress in your life (e.g., fears, concerns, expectations)?

Do you have any allergies?

When did you last eat?

PAST MEDICAL HISTORY

Do any of the following apply to you?

- known kidney, gall bladder, or ovarian disease
- history of urinary tract infections
- abdominal surgery
- episodes of bowel obstruction
- trauma
- coronary artery disease

What medications do you take (e.g., anticoagulants, NSAIDs, steroids)?

Have you had any STDs?

Do any diseases run in your family (e.g., inflammatory bowel disease)?

Female patients:

- When was your last menstrual period? How regular are your periods?
- Do you have vaginal discharge or pain with intercourse?
- Have you ever been pregnant? If so, how many times? How many children do you have? Did you have any complications during delivery?

What type of contraception do you use?

How many sexual partners do you have?

Do you drink alcohol? How much, how often?

Do you use recreational drugs?

Physical exam

CATEGORY TO ASSESS	DETAILS
General appearance	Assess: LOC, ABCs, vitals, position, nutritional status
	Assess for:
	• dehydration, jaundice, anemia
	• cyanosis, cardiorespiratory distress
	• septic appearance
	• stigmata of liver disease: spider nevi, palmar erythema, ascites, muscle wasting, gynecomastia, testicular atrophy, caput medusa, asterixis
	• peripheral edema
	• leukonychia, koilonychias

(Continued)

CATEGORY TO ASSESS	DETAILS
Chest	Chest: look for splinting, pleural friction rub, consolidation, chest wall tenderness
	Heart: listen for heart murmur, extra heart sounds, crackles (heart failure symptoms)
Abdomen	Inspection:
	• peristalsis
	• scars (previous surgeries), striae
	• hernia (umbilical, inguinal)
	• distension
	• Cullen sign: periumbilical blue discoloration due to retroperitoneal hemorrhage
	• Grey-Turner sign: bluish flank discoloration due to retroperitoneal hemorrhage
	Palpation:
	• light palpation for pain, deep for mass
	• liver, spleen, kidney, bladder, aorta
	• pulsatile mass with bruit: AAA
	• peritoneal signs: Rovsing sign, psoas, obturator, shake tenderness, cough tenderness
	• pain at McBurney point
	• Kehr sign: left shoulder pain from splenic rupture
	• Blumberg sign: rebound
	• Courvoisier sign: palpable tender gallbladder (pancreatic cancer)
	• Murphy sign: inspiratory arrest on deep palpation of right upper quadrant (RUQ) due to cholecystitis
	Percussion:
	• liver margin, spleen (in Traube space)
	• costal vertebral angle
	• shifting dullness/percussion, dullness/percussion wave for ascites
	• suprapubic dullness
	Auscultation:
	• bowel sounds
	• aortic and renal bruits
	• hepatic and splenic rubs
Inguinal region	Look for hernias
	Inspect and palpate testicles
Rectum Female patients: vagina	Examine: rectal mucosa, prostate, uterus
	Look for adnexal masses, cervical motion tenderness, adnexal tenderness, vaginal discharge/bleeding

Differential diagnosis

Etiologies for pain in the lower left quadrant (LLQ) include:

- diverticulitis
- ureteral stone (renal colic)
- ectopic pregnancy
- pelvic inflammatory disease/tubo-ovarian abscess
- ovarian torsion, torsion of ovarian cyst
- appendicitis
- mittelschmerz
- irritable bowel syndrome
- inflammatory bowel disease
- chronic pain syndromes

Etiologies for flank pain include:

- kidney stone
- renal infarction
- pyelonephritis
- spinal or paraspinal muscle spasm
- renal stone (suggested by family history of renal stone, cystinuria, uric acid, renal tubular acidosis, hyperparathyroidism, milk-alkali syndrome, bone metastases)

Investigations

Recommend, as appropriate:

- CBC, differential
- abdominal series, CXR
- beta-hCG
- paracentesis, peritoneal lavage
- US
- electrolytes, BUN, Cr, amylase, bilirubin, LFTs, blood C&S
- urinalysis C&S
- stool for ova and parasites
- CT abdomen/pelvis
- barium enema/upper GI endoscopy, IVP, ERCP

Case 109: Acute severe abdominal pain

A 40-year-old man comes to the emergency room with agonizing abdominal pain. Please carry out the necessary examination and provide a differential diagnosis. Initiate appropriate management.

Time: 5 minutes

Physical exam

Talk to the patient for more information and give a running commentary as you do the exam.

Assess:

- ABCs
- vitals, BP sitting and supine

Pay attention to signs of shock: BP 90/60 and pulse rate more than 100.

Perform an abdominal exam: check for rebound tenderness, peritoneal signs (pancreatitis or perforated bowel).

Differential diagnosis

Etiologies for severe abdominal pain include:

- acute pancreatitis (history of binge drinking and gastritis)
- perforated duodenal ulcer
- acute cholecystitis
- renal colic
- ovarian torsion
- spinal or paraspinal muscle spasm
- bowel obstruction

Management

Start: IV NS 1L over 30 minutes.

Attach/insert: NG tube, Foley catheter, oxygen, cardiac monitor.

Initiate investigations:

- CBC, type and crossmatch, electrolytes, BUN, Cr, Ca, amylase
- abdominal X-ray, US, CT

Do a general surgery consult.

After the surgery consult, administer analgesia: meperidine 50 mg IV.

Case 110: Thyroid mass

A middle-aged woman presents with a thyroid mass. Please obtain a history, do a focused physical exam, and recommend investigations.

Time: 5 minutes

History

Be aware of possible indicators of malignancy: voice change, rapid growth, no response to levothyroxine therapy, positive family history, history of radiation.

HISTORY OF PRESENT ILLNESS

When did you notice the mass? Has it changed since you noticed it?

Does the mass move with swallowing?

Do you have any difficulty or discomfort with breathing or swallowing?

Is the mass painful?

Have there been any changes in your voice?

Do you have any other neck lumps?

Do you have any of the following symptoms?

- heat intolerance, irritability, fine tremor, palpitations, diarrhea (symptoms of hyperthyroidism)
- fatigue, cold intolerance, mental/physical slowing, constipation (symptoms of hypothyroidism)

PAST MEDICAL HISTORY

Have you ever been treated with levothyroxine for thyroid cancer? Did your thyroid shrink?

Have you ever received radiation on your neck or head?

Does your family have a history of thyroid cancer?

Physical exam

Pay attention to features that indicate malignancy: diffuse enlargement versus nodules in the thyroid, the character of nodules, regional lymphadenopathy.

Palpate the thyroid at rest and with swallowing. Assess the mobility of the thyroid/mass.

Palpate the cervical lymph nodes.

Investigations

As appropriate, recommend:

- US
- thyroid function tests: TSH, free thyroxine (T4)
- thyroid scan
- fine needle aspiration

Case 111: Ankle sprain

A 20-year-old man presents with an ankle injury. Please assess the injury, recommend investigations, and initiate appropriate management.

Time: 5 minutes

Assessment of injury

Ask the patient: What was the position of the ankle or foot at the time of the injury?

Determine what motion relates to the injury: supination-adduction, supination-eversion (external rotation), pronation-abduction, or pronation-eversion.

Localize the tenderness, swelling, ecchymosis, and deformity. Determine if the patient has any bone pain.

Perform key tests: anterior drawer test, passive inversion.

Investigations

Apply the Ottawa ankle rules (see Table 33). Recommend, as appropriate:

- X-ray: posterior/anterior, lateral, mortise

Table 33. OTTAWA ANKLE RULES*

WHAT TO X-RAY	WHEN TO X-RAY
Ankle	Bone pain plus one of the following: • medial malleolus tenderness • lateral malleolus tenderness • inability to bear weight for 4 steps both immediately after injury and in the emergency room

(Continued)

Table 33. (*Continued*)

WHAT TO X-RAY	WHEN TO X-RAY
Foot	Bone pain plus one of the following: • tenderness of fifth metatarsal base • navicular tenderness • inability to bear weight for 4 steps both immediately after injury and in the emergency room

* Adapted from Stiell IG, Greenberg GH, McKnight RD, Nair RC, McDowell I, Worthington JR. A study to develop clinical decision rules for the use of radiography in acute ankle injuries. *Ann Emerg Med.* 1992;21(4):384–90. PMID 1554175.

Management

Manage according to the severity of the injury (see Table 34).

Table 34. ANKLE SPRAIN SEVERITY

CATEGORY	INJURY
First degree	Stretched ligament fibers
Second degree	Partial tear with pain and swelling
Third degree	Complete ligament separation

Remember (mnemonic: **RICE**): **r**est, **i**ce, **c**ompression, **e**levation.

Counsel the patient about immediate steps to control swelling:

- Wrap the ankle in an elastic bandage.
- Apply an ice pack, or immerse the ankle in ice water, for 15 to 20 minutes every 3 to 4 hours for 48 hours.
- When awake, elevate the foot and take analgesics.

For a first or second degree sprain, the patient needs to take the following steps:

- Stop ice and change to hot soak after 48 hours.
- Continue wrapping the ankle in an elastic bandage for 1 to 2 weeks (wrapped ankle should be in a neutral or slightly outward position).
- Use a crutch and allow only partial weight bearing until the ankle has no pain.
- Begin non-weight-bearing exercise in 2 to 3 days, including flexing the foot up and down, moving the foot from side to side, and flexing the toes.
- After the pain and swelling subside, use a sprain brace (as needed for pain control) and allow full weight bearing.

For a third degree sprain, the patient needs the following steps:

- surgical repair
- cast immobilization for 4 to 8 weeks
- referral to orthopedics

Case 112: Abdominal injury

A 20-year-old man has been stabbed in the epigastrium. His blood pressure reading is 90/40. Please initiate appropriate management.

Time: 5 minutes

Management

PRIMARY SURVEY

Ensure ABCs.

Pay attention to color (pale, cyanotic), sweating, respiratory distress (more than 36 breaths/min), agitation.

If airway and breathing are intact, check vitals. Check femoral pulse if the patient has no palpable radial pulse.

Establish IV access: 2 large bore IVs running a crystalloid; rate depends on clinical situation. If more than 2 L required for treatment of shock, consider blood transfusion.

SECONDARY SURVEY

Ask the patient: What happened? How do you feel? Where is the pain?

Do a physical exam (see breakdown that follows).

CATEGORY TO ASSESS	DETAILS
Abdomen	Assess:
	• local and rebound tenderness
	• wound assessment
	• bowel sounds
	• distension
Chest	Assess:
	• both sides of chest for movement
	• breath sound (pneumothorax, hemothorax)
	• heart sounds (tamponade)

(*Continued*)

CATEGORY TO ASSESS	DETAILS
Rectum	Perform DRE, vaginal exam
Female patients: vagina	Assess:
	• bleeding
	• perforation

Recheck ABCs.

Insert NG tube and Foley catheter (unless there is blood at meatus indicating urethral injury).

Initiate investigations: CBC, type and screen, electrolytes, urinalysis.

Specify nothing by mouth (npo) in anticipation of surgery; administer IV analgesia.

Consult surgery.

Case 113: Fall and trauma

A 30-year-old man has fallen from a height of 10 meters. He presents with tenderness in the left upper quadrant (LUQ) and a wound on the left leg. He has a neck collar on but wants it removed. He wants analgesics. Please initiate appropriate management.

Time: 10 minutes

Management

PRIMARY SURVEY

Ensure ABCs.

Take C-spine precautions.

Administer 100% oxygen.

Start 2 large bore IVs. Administer IV hydration. Type and screen blood in anticipation of transfusion.

SECONDARY SURVEY

Get incident details from the patient and from family, friends, witnesses, etc. Ask about:

- height of fall
- how the patient landed
- loss of consciousness/amnesia

Take a mini history (mnemonic: **AMPLE**):

- **a**llergies
- **m**edications
- **p**ast medical history
- **l**ast eaten
- **e**vents leading to condition

Perform a physical exam:

- Assess ABCs, vitals. (Note: low blood pressure could be due to blood loss or spinal cord injury.)
- Look for medical alert tags, bracelets, necklace.
- Do a head-to-toe survey.
- Assess spine for:
  - tenderness over spinous processes
  - paraspinal swelling
  - gap between spinous processes (interspinous ligament rupture)
- Assess for urinary retention, priapism, urinary/fecal incontinence.
- Perform a DRE.
- Do an abdominal exam.

Requisition 3 X-rays: C-spine (anterior/posterior, lateral, odontoid views), chest, pelvis.

Do a neurologic exam: LOC (see Table 25), focal signs, numbness/immobility in limbs.

Deal with problems in order of importance (see breakdown that follows).

CATEGORY	DETAILS
C-spine	Clear if:
	• no pain, no tenderness, no neurological signs/symptoms
	• no significant distracting injury
	• no head injury
	• no intoxication
	• normal X-rays
	Requisition CT if:
	• abnormal X-rays
	• neurological findings

(*Continued*)

CATEGORY	DETAILS
Spleen	Clear if:
	• vitals stable and no peritoneal signs
	If unstable, requisition (mnemonic: **FAST**):
	• **f**ocused **a**bdominal **s**onography in **t**rauma
Wound	Assess for and manage nerve, vessel, and tendon damage
	Consult plastics as needed
	Clean and suture wound
	Administer, as appropriate:
	• tetanus toxoid
	• antibiotics
Analgesia	Patient can have low dose narcotics if:
	• vitals stable
	• LOC normal
	• clear C-spine

Monitor the patient closely.

If the patient is admitted, perform a full head-to-toe survey the next day for missed injuries (tertiary survey).

Case 114: Head trauma

A patient has suffered a head trauma in a motor vehicle collision. Please initiate appropriate management.

Time: 10 minutes

Management

As you manage the patient, keep the following in mind:

- Never do a lumbar puncture.
- Always consider C-spine injury.
- Don't assume a coma is alcohol induced.
- Low BP indicates an injury unless proven otherwise.
- Avoid overhydration (cerebral edema).

PRIMARY SURVEY

Ensure ABCs:

- For airway: immobilize C-spine, and administer suction and inline traction for nasal or endotracheal tube.
- If the patient can talk, do not intubate; if unable to talk, intubate (no nasal tube if there is a major facial fracture).
- Administer 100% oxygen, elevate head of bed if thoracic and lumbar spines are cleared.
- Rule out (mnemonic: **ATOM CEF**): **a**irway obstruction, **t**ension/**o**pen pneumothorax, **m**assive hemothorax, **c**ardiac tamponade, **e**xsanguinous active bleeding, and **f**lail chest.
- Start 2 large bore IVs, NS or Ringer's lactate (RL) 2 L bolus.
- Start cardiac monitors.
- Maintain BP (thereby maintaining central perfusion pressure).

Differentiate hypotensive shock (low BP, high pulse) from neurogenic shock (low BP, low pulse).

Scan for obvious blood loss.

Insert NG tube, Foley catheter unless contraindicated.

Check vitals.

Initiate investigations: ECG, ABG, glucose, toxicity screen, blood type and screen.

Assess for spinal cord injury: weakness, numbness, spinal pain, LOC.

Initiate a neurosurgery consult.

SECONDARY SURVEY

Get details of the collision from the patient and from family, friends, witnesses, etc. Ask about:

- circumstances of the collision
- mechanism of the injury
  - whether the seat belt was on
  - where the patient was found
  - whether the patient hit the windshield
  - whether the patient was the driver
- loss of consciousness (How long?)
- posttraumatic amnesia
- loss of sensation/function

Take a mini history (mnemonic: **AMPLE**):

- **a**llergies
- **m**edications
- **p**ast medical history
- **l**ast eaten
- **e**vents leading to condition

Do a head-to-toe survey:

- Expose the patient to look for injuries. If the patient has a cervical collar, open it (if the patient is calm) to check C-spine and trachea.
- Check every orifice.
- Check for medical alert tags.
- Check for fractures.
- Look for specific toxidromes.
- Check (mnemonic: **5Ns**): **n**oggin ("raccoon eyes," Battle sign), **n**eck (C-spine), E**N**T (ear/nose/throat), **n**eedle (tracks for drug abuse), **n**eurological condition.

Do a neurological exam (see breakdown that follows).

CATEGORY	WHAT TO ASSESS/LOOK FOR
LOC	See Table 25
Head and neck	Lacerations, bruises, basal skull fracture, facial fractures, foreign bodies
Cerebrospinal fluid (CSF)	"Double ring" sign on a blotting paper (blood forms a circle, or "inner ring," surrounded by an outer ring of CSF)
Increased intracranial pressure	Hiccup, yawn, Cushing reflex (BP high, low pulse), breathing pattern, pupil size and reactivity, extraocular movements, nystagmus, fundoscopy
Brain stem injury	Cranial nerve palsies, breathing pattern, "doll's eyes"
Spine	Deformity, tenderness
Motor responses	Muscle tone, power, sensation, ability to move fingers/toes
	If unconscious, test reflexes (corneal, abdominal, sphincter, Achilles) and response to pain/stimulation (e.g., squeeze nail beds)

Initiate investigations:

- X-ray (assess alignment, bone, cartilage, and soft tissue): cervical, thoracic, and lumbar spine (anterior/posterior, lateral, odontoid: must see C1 to T1)
- CT: head and upper C-spine
- CXR, CBC, urine drug screen

FOLLOW-UP MANAGEMENT

For a minor head injury:

- Observe for 24 to 48 hours.
- Wake up every hour.
- Do not administer sedatives or painkillers.

For a severe head injury:

- Ensure ABCs, vitals, and neuro vitals.
- If increased intracranial pressure (ICP), administer mannitol 1 g/kg IV, followed by surgery, elevation of head, hyperventilation.
- Patient needs surgery to evacuate hematoma (do a neurosurgery consult).

For a spinal injury:

- Reduce dislocation by traction or surgery, and stabilize.
- Emergency surgical decompression and/or fusion may be required.

Continued care:

- Continue evaluation and therapy, and consults with various surgical subspecialties, as indicated.
- Work out appropriate disposition (home, admission, admission to ICU) depending on the clinical situation.

Case 115: Suturing of laceration

A 20-year-old man has lacerated his right forearm on a broken beer bottle. Please obtain a history, do a physical exam, and initiate appropriate management.

Time: 10 minutes

History

HISTORY OF PRESENT ILLNESS

When did the injury happen?

Where were you?

What caused the injury (e.g., knife, falling object)? What was its position, direction, and power?

Was there visible arterial spurting at the time of injury?

Do any of the following apply to you?

- associated injuries
- dizziness
- head trauma
- headache

PAST MEDICAL HISTORY

Have you had any previous hand trauma or surgery?

Do you have any allergies?

What medications are you taking?

Have you had tetanus shots? How many? When?

Which is your dominant hand?

What is your occupation? What do you do for recreation (e.g., sports, hobbies)?

Physical exam

Ensure ABCs, hemodynamic stability.

Follow these general considerations in wound management:

- Consider every structure deep to a laceration severed until proven otherwise.
- Test nerve function against resistance.
- Do not test tendon function against resistance.

- Examine tendon function and neurovascular status distal to the injury.
- X-ray for foreign bodies if necessary.
- Clean and explore wounds under local anesthetic.

Inspect: deformity, depth and range of laceration, active bleeding, color (pale, blue), swelling, bruising, perfusion.

Palpate: pulse, temperature, sensation.

Assess ROM: be careful, don't test function against resistance.

Assess damaged structures (see Table 35):

- nerve: sensory loss, motor (extrinsic/intrinsic muscles, superficial and deep), sympathetic system (sweating)
- vessels: capillary refill, Allen test, color, turgor, temperature
- tendon: don't test against resistance

Table 35. WRIST INJURIES: STRUCTURES THAT CAN BE SEVERED

CATEGORY	STRUCTURES
Superficial structures	Flexor carpi ulnaris, flexor carpi radialis, palmaris longus
Deep structures	Flexor digitorum superficialis and profundus, adductor pollicis longus
Nerves	Median nerve, ulnar nerve
Vessels	Radial artery, ulnar artery

Management

CATEGORY	MANAGEMENT
Nerve	Primary repair generally advocated, although delayed repair may have benefit in certain cases
	Refer to plastic surgery
Vessel	Control bleeding with direct pressure and hand elevation
	Avoid probing, clamping, or tying off to avoid nerve injury
	Suture
	Dress, immobilize, splint with fingertips visible
	Monitor: color, turgor, capillary refill, temperature
Tendon	Requires primary repair
	Never immobilize more than 3 weeks to avoid stiffness

PROCEDURE FOR SUTURING

Wash your hands, wear gloves.

Apply local anesthetic (avoid epinephrine in cases involving fingers, nose, toes, ears, or penis).

Irrigate copiously with NS.

Control bleeding with direct pressure. Do not clamp structures because of risk to nerves. Consult general/plastic surgery if necessary.

Prepare the field with iodine and sterile draping.

Debride dead tissue with a sharp instrument (scissors or scalpel). Remove foreign bodies.

Use absorbable sutures for subcutaneous tissue: catgut, Dexon, Vicryl.

Use plain catgut for small vessels and chromic catgut for large vessels. Plain catgut is absorbed more quickly than chromic.

Use nylon for skin: face 6-0, scalp 3-0 to 4-0, trunk 4-0 to 5-0, joint 4-0 to 5-0. Make sutures 2 to 3 mm apart, 2 to 3 mm from edge.

Apply splinting, or internal/external fixation, for fractures and for anastomosis of important vessels and nerves.

Dress the wound. The dressing can be removed after 24 hours and the patient can shower in 1 to 2 days.

Administer tetanus prophylaxis (see Table 36).

Table 36. TETANUS PROPHYLAXIS

IMMUNIZATION HISTORY	NONTETANUS-PRONE WOUNDS		TETANUS-PRONE WOUNDS*	
	TD**	TIG***	TD	TIG
Uncertain or < 3 doses	yes	no	yes	yes
3 or more doses, but none for more than 10 years	yes	no	yes	no
3 or more doses in the last 5–10 years	no	no	yes	no
3 or more doses in the last 4 years	no	no	no	no

* wounds more than 6 hours old, more than 1 cm deep that are puncture wounds, avulsions, wounds resulting from missiles, crush wounds, burns, frostbite, or contaminated with dirt, soil, saliva

** tetanus/diphtheria

*** tetanus immunoglobulin

Administer antibiotics:

- topical antibiotic ointment for superficial wounds (patient to use as needed)
- systemic if laceration penetrated bone, tendon, or joint space

Recheck circulation, nerve (sensation, motor) after suturing.

Follow these guidelines for suture removal:

- joint: 14–21 days
- face: 3–5 days
- oral mucosa: 10–14 days
- scalp 5–7 days
- other sites: 7 days

Case 116: Burns

A burn victim comes to the emergency room. Please initiate appropriate management.

Time: 10 minutes

Management

PRIMARY SURVEY

Ensure ABCs.

Assess need for oxygen or hyperbaric oxygen by measuring carboxy hemoglobin (ABG sample).

Ensure the burning process has stopped: remove the patient's clothes.

Monitor airway and breathing for upper airway edema.

For circulation:

- Start 2 large bore IVs in an upper extremity: go through burned skin if necessary.
- Patients with burns to more than 20% of total body surface area (TBSA) need IV support.

SECONDARY SURVEY

Calculate TBSA burned (mnemonic: **rule of 9s**):

- each arm: 9%
- face/scalp: 9%

- back: 18%
- front: 18%
- each leg: 18%
- perineum: 1%
- patient's own hand area: 1%

Observe for inhalation injury. Factors suggesting inhalation injury include:

- confined in a burning building
- explosion
- loss of consciousness
- carbon deposits around nose, mouth, throat, in sputum
- inflammatory changes in oropharynx
- change in voice
- curled/singed facial hair

Perform a head-to-toe examination:

- Look for other injuries.
- Remove jewelry to prevent circulatory compromise, escharotomy, or fasciotomy.

Assess ongoing needs for IV fluid support:

- Parkland formula: 4 cc × % TBSA burned × weight in kg
- half given in the first 8 hours after the burn injury
- half given in the subsequent 16 hours

Treat pain and prevent secondary infection:

- pain control
- systemic antibiotics
- wound care: cover with sterile dressing, topical silver sulfadiazine, antibiotic ointment for face
- tetanus prophylaxis

Case 117: Testicular pain

An 18-year-old man is experiencing testicular pain. Please take a focused history, do a focused physical exam, provide a differential diagnosis, and recommend investigations.

Time: 5 minutes

History

When did the pain start?

How rapidly did the pain develop?

Was the pain preceded by any of the following?

- trauma
- fever or swelling of the salivary glands (i.e., mumps)

Have you experienced any urinary changes (burning, discharge)?

Is the pain associated with a deformity or lump?

Do you have a history of the following?

- testicular trauma or surgery
- testicular disease

Physical exam

Assess the testicles for temperature, swelling, erythema.

Palpate for pain and for nodules/lumps.

Check for "blue dot" sign (torsion of epididymal appendage).

Differential diagnosis

Possible etiologies of testicular pain include:

- trauma
- infection (mumps, orchitis)
- epididymitis
- testicular torsion
- torsion of epididymal cyst
- torsion of epididymal appendage

Investigations

Recommend an emergent Doppler US to rule out torsion.

Case 118: Hernia

A 60-year-old man says he has a bulge in the groin. Please take a history, do a physical exam, recommend investigations, and outline a management plan.

Time: 5 minutes

History

How long have you had the bulge?

Has it changed in size?

Does anything make the bulge better or worse (e.g., relief with lying supine, pain with pressure or increased intraabdominal pressure)?

Are you experiencing vomiting, constipation, or a feeling of fullness? (Assess for obstructive factors.)

Do any of the following apply to you?

- obesity
- chronic cough
- straining
- heavy lifting
- female patients: pregnancy

Physical exam

Assess:

- location of hernia (internal, external, femoral, incisional, etc.)
- reducibility
- presence of bowel contents

Investigations

Recommend US.

Management

The patient needs:

- a hernia truss
- surgical repair for incarcerated/strangulated hernias and to avoid incarceration

Case 119: Breast lump

A 60-year-old woman presents with a breast lump. Please obtain a history, recommend investigations, and provide appropriate management.

Time: 5 minutes

History

HISTORY OF PRESENT ILLNESS

When did you find the lump? Do you do regular breast exams?

Have you noticed any changes in the size or mobility of the mass?

Do you have any of the following?

- nipple discharge
- nodes in the areas surrounding the breast (axilla)
- changes in the skin of the breast (e.g., skin tethering)

PAST MEDICAL HISTORY

Do you have a family history of breast cancer?

Have you had any of the following?

- previous breast biopsy or trauma, or benign breast disease
- previous low dose breast irradiation
- ovarian or endometrial cancer

Are you taking hormone replacement therapy?

How old were you when you had your first period? (Or—as appropriate— when your breasts began to develop?)

Do you drink alcohol? How much, how often?

Do you smoke?

Investigations

Recommend, as appropriate:

- mammogram
- fine needle aspiration (FNA), core needle biopsy, excisional biopsy/ lumpectomy (as appropriate)

Management

Advise the patient about common causes of breast lumps, as appropriate:

- younger than 35: fibrocystic change, fibroadenoma, bacterial mastitis, carcinoma (uncommon), fat necrosis (rare)
- 35 to 50 years old: fibrocystic change, carcinoma, fibroadenoma, mastitis, fat necrosis
- 50 years old: carcinoma, fibrocystic change, fat necrosis, mastitis

Discuss treatments, as appropriate, with the patient:

- surgical: breast conserving surgery versus mastectomy
- radiation
- chemotherapy
- hormone therapy in estrogen- or progesterone-receptor positive tumors (tamoxifen)
- prophylactic tamoxifen or mastectomy in high risk patients

Counsel the patient to consider genetic screening if the patient has:

- breast and ovarian cancer
- a strong family history of breast or ovarian cancer, or male breast cancer

Case 120: Prostate cancer

A 60-year-old man has been unable to urinate for 12 hours. Please obtain a history, provide a differential diagnosis, and recommend investigations.

Time: 5 minutes

History

HISTORY OF PRESENT ILLNESS

Is this a new problem or an ongoing problem?

When did the problem start?

How has it changed since it began?

Does anything make it better or worse (e.g., alcohol, spicy food)?

Do you have any of the following?

- blood in your urine
- fecal incontinence, loss of sensation in the perineum
- incontinence, burning, dysuria, hesitancy, trouble initiating stream
- abdominal pain, fever, cough, backache, weight loss, loss of appetite, decreased energy level
- leg or facial swelling
- back pain

How frequently do you have to urinate? Has this changed over time? Do you need to urinate overnight?

PAST MEDICAL HISTORY

Have you ever had back surgery or spinal trauma?

Do you have any allergies?

What medications do you take?

Do you have a family history of prostate cancer?

Have you had any STDs?

What is the pattern of your sexual activity? (Assess risk for STDs.)

Do you drink, smoke, or take recreational drugs?

Differential diagnosis

Possible etiologies of urinary retention in men include:

- prostate cancer
- BPH

- cauda equina syndrome
- urethral obstruction (valve, stricture)

Investigations

Recommend:

- DRE, prostate-specific antigen (PSA), transrectal US and biopsy
- urinalysis, urine cytology
- bone scan, CT (if cancer found on biopsy)

Management

Treatment for BPH includes:

- alpha-adrenergic antagonist (terazosin) to reduce prostate muscle tone
- 5-alpha reductase inhibitor to reduce prostate size
- surgery: TURP, open prostatectomy, other stents, microwave, laser therapy, etc.

Treatment for prostate cancer includes:

- stage T1, T2: radical surgery
- stage T3, T4: staging adenectomy, radiation, hormone therapy, orchiectomy, luteinizing hormone-releasing hormone (LH-RH) agonist (e.g., leuprolide acetate)

Case 121: Lower GI bleeding

A patient presents with lower GI bleeding. Please take a history, give a differential diagnosis, and initiate appropriate management.

Time: 5 minutes

History

Before you begin the history, assess the patient for hemodynamic instability: vitals, chest pain, diaphoresis, confusion, tachypnea, pallor, shortness of breath. Stabilize the patient immediately, if necessary.

HISTORY OF PRESENT ILLNESS

How much blood are you losing? How long have you had the bleeding?

Is it bright red blood or dark blood?

Do you see the blood smeared on stools, mixed into stools, on wiping, or in your underwear?

Do any of the following apply to you?

- recent intense retching
- taking iron pills or bismuth (Rule out pseudobleed.)
- diet rich in leafy green vegetables

Do you have any of the following symptoms?

- nausea and vomiting
- vomiting blood
- abdominal pain
- diarrhea, constipation, black/tarry feces
- weight loss
- abdominal cramps

PAST MEDICAL HISTORY

Do you have a history of any of the following?

- hemorrhoids
- constipation
- inflammatory bowel disease
- liver disease
- coagulation disorders

Are you taking any of the following medications?

- warfarin
- heparin

- NSAIDs
- steroids

Differential diagnosis

Etiologies for lower GI bleeding include:

- diverticulosis
- angiodysplasia
- hemorrhoid
- inflammatory bowel disease
- colon cancer
- coagulation disorder
- vasculitis
- liver cirrhosis
- NSAID or steroid use
- alcohol abuse
- peptic or duodenal ulcer
- Mallory-Weiss syndrome
- diverticulosis

Management

In severe cases of bleeding, ensure ABCs and stabilize.

Perform a sigmoidoscopy on unprepared bowel.

- Diagnostic results include: bleeding hemorrhoids, colitis, structural lesion. Treat accordingly.
- If the results are nondiagnostic, hospitalize.
  o If the bleeding stops, clean the bowel and do a colonoscopy.
  o If still bleeding:
    - < 0.5 mL/min, then RBC scan
    - 0.5 mL/min, then angiogram

Case 122: Vomiting

An adult patient presents with vomiting of several days duration. Please take a focused history.

Time: 5 minutes

History

HISTORY OF PRESENT ILLNESS

How long has the vomiting been occurring?

Are there any triggers (e.g., is it worse in the morning or after meals)?

Do you have any of the following?

- abdominal pain or headache
- bloody or bile-stained vomit
- recognizable food or bright red blood in the vomit
- vomit that looks like coffee grounds
- gastroesophageal reflux (heartburn, regurgitation into the mouth)
- urination, or concentrated urine

Are you tolerating fluids?

PAST MEDICAL HISTORY

What medications do you take?

Do you drink alcohol? How much, how often?

Do you use recreational drugs?

Case 123: Constipation

A 50-year-old woman says she is experiencing chronic constipation. Please take a focused history and suggest investigations.

Time: 5 minutes

History

HISTORY OF PRESENT ILLNESS

How long have you had this problem?

What characterizes your constipation?

What is your normal stool frequency?

Do you strain when you have a bowel movement?

Are the stools large, or small and pellet shaped?

Do you have abdominal pain, nausea, vomiting, or abdominal bloating?

Does the constipation alternate with periods diarrhea?

What is your usual diet (breakfast, lunch, supper)?

How much fiber do you eat?

PAST MEDICAL HISTORY

Do you have a history of spinal injury, abdominal or spinal surgery, or gastrointestinal tumor?

What medications do you take (i.e., opiates, neuroleptics, or antidepressants)?

Do you use laxatives? How often and what type?

Investigations

Recommend:

- rectal and perineal examination to look for tumors or evidence of an inflammatory process
- CBC to look for anemia, which could indicate bowel cancer
- fecal occult blood
- abdominal X-ray

Consider colonoscopy (if the patient is over 50), after constipation has been relieved, to rule out bowel cancer.

Case 124: Diarrhea

A 70-year-old woman has had diarrhea since discharge from hospital 10 days ago. Please take a focused history and suggest investigations.

Time: 5 minutes

History

HISTORY OF PRESENT ILLNESS

How long have you had diarrhea?

How many times per day are you having a bowel movement?

What is your normal stool frequency?

Are you awakened with a bowel movement at night?

Is there any blood, pus, or mucous present in the diarrhea?

What color is the diarrhea?

Do any of the following apply to you?

- nausea and vomiting, weight loss, or cramping
- thirst, dizziness, decreased urination
- recent travel outside the country
- contact with people who have diarrhea

Have you eaten any undercooked meats recently (e.g., hamburgers) or contaminated produce?

Have you eaten at a restaurant recently?

PAST MEDICAL HISTORY

Do you have a history of any bowel diseases (e.g. inflammatory bowel disease)?

What medications are you taking (e.g., antibiotics)?

Do you use laxatives? How often and what type?

What is your sexual orientation?

Have you had any unprotected sex?

Investigations

The patient's history of recent hospitalization should trigger concern for *Clostridium difficile*. Order stool for *C. difficile*.

Additional testing is usually not warranted unless the patient has other risk factors or chronic diarrhea.

Consider stool cultures if the patient is immunocompromised or is a food handler.

Consider endoscopy if there is concern about inflammatory bowel disease, ischemic colitis, or microscopic colitis.

Case 125: Upper GI bleeding

A patient presents with hematemesis. Please initiate appropriate management.

Time: 5 minutes

Management

PRIMARY SURVEY

Ensure ABCs. If the patient is in a coma, intubate.

Administer oxygen supplementation.

Start 2 large bore IVs, ensure hemodynamic stability, and give crystalloid, plasma, or blood as needed.

The patient should have nothing by mouth (npo).

Insert NG tube to see if the bleeding is from an upper GI source. If so, empty the stomach and insert a balloon tamponade.

Monitor urine output.

Initiate investigations:

- type and screen blood (crossmatch 6 to 10 units of blood)
- CBC, Cr, electrolytes, urea
- PTT, INR
- ECG monitor
- CXR

Hold all anticoagulants and NSAIDs.

Administer:

- fluids if hypotension
- oxygen

- morphine for pain
- pantoprazole infusion

Do a GI consult for endoscopy.

SECONDARY SURVEY

During the secondary survey, make sure the bleeding is from a GI source.

Note that:

- Hematemesis usually indicates bleeding site proximal to Treitz ligament.
- Vomiting fresh red blood suggests continuous bleeding. It also allows a rough estimate of the rate of bleeding. If the blood stays in the stomach for any substantial amount of time, it will look like coffee grounds.
- Bleeding sufficient to produce hematemesis usually results in melena. Less than half of patients with melena have hematemesis.
- Sharp, burning, or gnawing pain that is relieved with food or antacids indicates peptic ulcer disease.

Take a history (see breakdown that follows).

HISTORY CATEGORY	QUESTIONS
History of present illness	When did you begin vomiting blood? How much? Has the problem changed in any way?
	Do you have pain? Where? Does it radiate to other parts of your body? Does anything make the pain better or worse?
	Were you vomiting before the bloody vomit started?
	Does it feel like blood is trickling down the back of your throat? (Assess for possible nosebleed.)
	What does the vomit look like? What is the color? Are there any clots?
	Have you had a bowel movement? What does your stool look like?
	Do you have any of the following symptoms?
	• recent weight loss
	• recent stomach discomfort
Past medical history	Do you have a history of illnesses (e.g., coagulopathy, atrial fibrillation, past pulmonary embolus, ulcers, varices, liver disease, protracted vomiting, loss of appetite, H. pylori)?
	Have you ever had an endoscopy?
	Have you had surgery or treatment for ulcer?
	What medications do you take (e.g., anticoagulants, aspirin, NSAIDs)?
	Do you drink or smoke?

Do a physical exam. Assess:

- vital signs: tachycardia, orthostatic hypotension, general appearance (pallor, diaphoresis, cool skin)

- HEENT: jugular venous pressure, mucous membrane moisture
- mouth and nasopharynx: rule out nonintestinal bleeding source
- stigmata of chronic liver disease: spider anima, gynecomastia, testicular atrophy, jaundice, ascites, hepatosplenomegaly
- abdomen: tenderness, mass lesion, guarding, rebound tenderness
- pedal edema
- rectum: color of stool, confirm fecal occult blood test (FOBT) positive

Treatment

Consult gastroenterologist for endoscopy and definitive treatment.

For peptic ulcer disease: cauterize visible vessels, inject epinephrine, administer triple therapy for *Helicobacter pylori* (clarithromycin, metronidazole, proton pump inhibitor).

For gastritis: treat *H. pylori* or other agents (alcohol, NSAIDS, etc.).

For varices: treat with endoscopic banding or injection of sclerosing agent, administer beta-blockers.

For Mallory-Weiss syndrome: consult general surgery if necessary.

Case 126: Lung nodule

A routine chest X-ray reveals a nodule in a 50-year-old female patient. Please perform a focused physical exam, provide a differential diagnosis, and recommend investigations.

Time: 5 minutes

Physical exam

CATEGORY	DETAILS
Inspection	Distress: nasal flare, pursed lip breathing, accessory muscle use
	Posture: sitting upright, use of pillows
	Chest shape: barrel chest, kyphosis, scoliosis, pectus excavatum, flail
	Skin: telangiectasia, cyanosis (central/peripheral), nicotine stain, cachexia, jaundice
Palpation	Lymph nodes: sub/supraclavicular and axillary area
	Mass and tenderness
	Tactile fremitus
	Trachea, breath excursions

(Continued)

CATEGORY	DETAILS
Percussion	Dull versus tympanic
	Diaphragmatic excursion
Auscultation	Air entry
	Wheeze, crackles
	Friction rub
	Audible bruit

Differential diagnosis

See Table 37.

Table 37. DIFFERENTIAL DIAGNOSIS OF LUNG NODULES

CATEGORY	POSSIBLE ETIOLOGY
Infection	Healed granuloma: TB, histoplasmosis, coccidiomycosis
Neoplasm	Benign: hamartoma
	Malignant: primary or metastatic (e.g., breast, colon, testicles)
Immune response	Sarcoidosis, amyloidosis
Congenital origin	Bronchogenic cyst, hydatid cyst, pseudolymphoma, arteriovenous malformation, bronchopulmonary sequestration
Extrapulmonary origin	Skin, nipple, chest wall, rib, pleural plaque

Factors that favor carcinoma include:

- speculated, irregular, or lobulated edge
- presence of other coin lesions
- associated mediastinal adenopathy or bony metastases
- growth compared to an earlier X-ray
- obstructive phenomenon (peripheral consolidation/atelectasis)

Factors that make carcinoma unlikely include:

- calcification
- cavity with darker center compared to circumference
- air fluid level (suggests abscess)

Investigations

Recommend:

- CBC, electrolytes, Cr
- CXR

- sputum culture, acid-fast bacilli (AFB), cytology
- CT/MRI
- bronchoscopy
- mediastinoscopy
- fine needle aspiration (FNA)

Case 127: Lung cancer

A 50-year-old smoker and current textile worker has a likely diagnosis of lung cancer. Please discuss a management plan with the patient.

Time: 5 minutes

Management

Ask the patient:

- What do you already know about your disease?
- What more would you like to know about your disease?
- What is on your mind?

Provide clear information about diagnosis, staging, and symptoms. Discuss possible cause.

Counsel the patient that there are major differences in prognosis based on tissue type and staging. Explain the prognosis for this particular patient.

Describe treatment options, as appropriate:

- nonsmall cell:
  - stage I/II: surgery
  - stage III: palliative
- small cell:
  - localized: surgery after radiation
  - extensive: chemotherapy, radiation

Form a treatment plan, respecting the patient's wishes.

Facilitate communication between the patient and the patient's family.

Case 128: Shock and collapse

An 80-year-old woman is brought to the emergency room by her granddaughter. She is unconscious with a heart rate of 40 and a blood pressure reading of 80/40. Please initiate appropriate management and provide a differential diagnosis.

Time: 10 minutes

Management

PRIMARY SURVEY

Ensure ABCs:

- Clear the airway: look, listen, and feel for flow of air.
- Check for breathing.
- Check pulses.

Initiate emergency management:

- Start 100% oxygen on 5 L.
- Establish 2 large bore IVs (at least 16-gauge).
- Consider fluid 1–2 L bolus.
- Type, screen, and crossmatch blood.
- Prepare for transcutaneous pacemaker.

Consider atropine 0.5 mg IV; consider epinephrine infusion (2–10 µg/min) or dopamine infusion (2–10 µg/kg/min).

Insert Foley catheter for urine output.

Attach ECG.

Check vitals q15min.

Initiate emergency cariology consult.

SECONDARY SURVEY

Do a physical exam (see breakdown that follows).

CATEGORY TO ASSESS	DETAILS
Neurological system	LOC (see Table 25), vision/hearing, cerebellar function/gait
Cardiovascular system	Orthostatic BP change, arrhythmia, murmurs, carotid bruits

(Continued)

CATEGORY TO ASSESS	DETAILS
Musculoskeletal system	Injury, joints, ill-fitting shoes
Abdomen	AAA
Extremities	Microcirculation in hands/feet

Initiate investigations: glucose, PTT, INR, BUN, Cr, ABG, CXR, troponin.

Get a history from family, friends, witnesses, paramedics, police, etc. Ask about:

- what the patient was doing at the time of the fall
- precipitating factors or warning signs before collapse
- health previous to collapse
- color of the patient during the event (red or pale)
- how quickly the patient recovered
- what medications the patient is taking
- previous similar episodes
- shortness of breath, chest pain, fever
- issues with shoes, joints, or with vision, hearing, or balance impairments

Differential diagnosis

Possible etiologies of shock and collapse include:

- cardiac event
  - arrhythmia: tachycardia (supraventricular tachycardia, atrial fibrillation, atrial flutter), bradycardia (sick sinus syndrome)
  - MI
  - obstruction: valvular, right ventricular outflow (pulmonary embolus)
  - CHF
- peripheral vascular event
  - hemorrhage
  - hypovolemia
  - anaphylaxis
- neurological event
  - seizure
  - migraine
  - cerebrovascular accident/TIA
- vasovagal event
- hyperventilation
- psychogenic event

Case 129: Hematuria

A routine urinalysis on a 50-year-old man reveals an RBC count of 50. Please take a history, perform a physical exam, provide a differential diagnosis, and recommend investigations.

Time: 10 minutes

History

HISTORY OF PRESENT ILLNESS

Can you see blood in your urine?

If yes:

- How much blood?
- Are there any clots?
- Which part of the urine stream is red: beginning, end, or throughout?

Do any of the following apply to you?

- painful urination
- changes in urinary frequency
- hesitancy in urination
- pelvic pain
- fever
- recent urinary tract infection
- changes in bowel habits or blood in your stools
- weight loss, night sweats
- recent changes in diet or medication (beets, dyes, rifampin)
- recent intense exercise or trauma
- for females: vaginal bleeding

Do you have back or side pain? (If yes, check onset, progression, and radiation.)

PAST MEDICAL HISTORY

Do you have a history of any of the following?

- coagulation disorder
- liver disease
- urinary tract infections

- bladder infections
- STDs
- TB
- kidney stones

What medications are you taking (e.g., anticoagulants, cancer treatments)?

Do you have a family history of polycystic disease, sickle cell disease, or early hearing loss?

For female patients:

- When was your last menstrual cycle?

Physical exam

Check:

- vitals
- skin: petechiae, ecchymosis, pallor
- HEENT
- chest: atrial fibrillation, valvular heart disease, costovertebral angle tenderness
- abdomen: enlarged renal masses (unilateral or bilateral), splenomegaly
- rectum: DRE for blood on finger, tender/boggy prostate
- overall: signs of trauma

Differential diagnosis

See Table 38.

Table 38. DIFFERENTIAL DIAGNOSIS OF HEMATURIA

CATEGORY	POSSIBLE ETIOLOGY
Transient	UTI, fever, endometriosis, thromboembolism, exercise, trauma
Renal	Tumor, glomerulopathy, vasculitis
Postrenal	Tumor, stone, papillary necrosis, cystitis, BPH, prostatitis
	Red urine (not blood)
	AAA

Etiology can also be classified as follows:

- painless hematuria
  - age 20 to 40: calculus
  - age 40 to 60: renal carcinoma
  - age 60 to 80: bladder carcinoma or BPH

- painful hematuria
  - UTI
  - stone
  - acute hemorrhagic cystitis
  - cyclophosphamide
  - AAA
- pseudohematuria
  - menses
  - hemoglobinuria
  - myoglobinuria
  - dyes (beets)
  - laxative
  - medications (rifampin)
  - porphyria
  - hematochezia
- less common
  - SLE
  - sickle cell disease
  - glomerulonephritis (GN)
  - intense exercise
  - masturbation

Investigations

Recommend, as appropriate:

- CBC: anemia, infection
- PTT, INR
- repeat urinalysis, 3 glass test, intravenous pyelogram
- renal function:
  - BUN, Cr, glomerular filtration rate (GFR)
  - 24 h protein-Cr ratio
- US kidneys, pelvis
- abdominal X-ray: kidney-ureter-bladder (KUB), flat plate, and upright
- further urology/nephrology consult:
  - cystoscopy, renal biopsy
  - immunologic studies: IgA, C3, C4, antistreptolysin O titer (ASOT)

Case 130: Neck and back pain

A patient is experiencing neck pain. Please take a history, perform a physical exam, provide a differential diagnosis, and outline a management plan.

Time: 10 minutes

History

HISTORY OF PRESENT ILLNESS

When did you start having neck pain?

Did it develop suddenly or gradually?

Do you know what triggered it?

If triggered by an injury:

- What was the nature of the injury?
- Did a noise in your neck accompany the injury?
- Were you able to walk afterwards?

Where is the maximal point of pain? Does the pain radiate to your limbs?

What is the pain like (e.g., throbbing, piercing)?

How severe is the pain on a scale of 1 (low) to 10 (high)?

Does anything make the pain better or worse (e.g., standing or sitting, moving or resting, bending, coughing and sneezing, driving, lifting)?

Do you have any of the following?

- numbness, weakness in limbs or perineum
- fever, weight loss
- morning stiffness
- bowel or bladder control issues
- current infections (sinuses, throat, ears)

PAST MEDICAL HISTORY

Have you had similar pain before? Did you receive treatment? How did that go?

Do you have a history of any of the following?

- coronary artery disease
- angina
- meningitis
- previous back surgery
- lumbar puncture

Do you take high dose steroids?

Does your family have a history of back problems or cancer?

Are you experiencing stress in your life (e.g., home, work, finances)?

Physical exam

See Table 39 for a correspondence of motor functions to C-spine level.

Table 39. SUMMARY OF MOTOR FUNCTIONS BY C-SPINE LEVEL

LEVEL	MOTOR	SENSORY	REFLEX
C5	deltoid	axillary	middle deltoid – biceps
C6	biceps	1, 2 finger	brachioradialis – biceps
C7	triceps	3 finger	triceps
C8	digits	4, 5 finger	finger jerk

POSITION OF PATIENT	DETAILS
Standing	Inspect from side and from behind: protruding abdomen, hyperlordosis, loss of lordosis, scoliosis, kyphosis, asymmetry, muscle bulk
	Assess:
	• gait: walking on heels (L4-L5), toes (S1); check symmetry of gait
	• squat (L2, L3, L4)
	• ROM: spine flexion/extension, internal/external rotation, lateral bending
	Palpate: spinal, paraspinal, and pelvic structures
	Measure occiput-to-wall distance, chest expansion
Sitting	Assess:
	• straight-leg raise (sciatica)
	• flexing knee, then straightening it to 90 degrees
	• reflexes: knee (L4) and ankle (S1)
	• costovertebral tenderness
Supine	Examine abdomen: inspect, palpate, percuss, auscultate
	Examine vascular system:
	• femoral, popliteal, dorsalis pedis, posterior tibial pulses
	• size, symmetry, swelling, pigmentation, ulcers
	• inguinal nodes, edema
	Assess sensory responses (with light touch, pin prick):
	• L4: anterior medial thigh and knee
	• L5: lateral leg, web space
	• S1: lateral heel, foot and toe

(Continued)

POSITION OF PATIENT	DETAILS
Supine (continued)	Assess motor responses (passive and active):
	• L4 (quads): extend knee against resistance
	• L5: dorsiflexion of great toe
	• S1: plantar flexion of foot
	Assess sacroiliac (SI) joint: Faber test
	Assess hip: ROM
Prone	Assess:
	• sensory responses for S2–S4: anal wink
	• sphincter tone
	• femoral stretch: L2, L4, hip and knee in extension
	• S1 (gluteus maximus): backward lift of leg against resistance

Differential diagnosis

CATEGORY	POSSIBLE ETIOLOGY
Surgical	Mild: muscle strain, ligament sprain, facet syndesis, degenerative disease, spondylolisthesis
	Moderate: sciatica/herniated disc, spinal stenosis
	Emergency: cauda equina syndrome (disc, mass, abscess, aortic aneurysm)
Medical	Neoplasm: multiple myeloma, osteoid osteoma
	Infectious: acute discitis, osteomyelitis, TB
	Inflammatory: ankylosing spondylitis, psoriatic spondylitis, reactive arthritis, inflammatory bowel disease
	Metabolic: osteoporosis, osteomalacia, Paget disease
	Viscera: endometriosis, pyelonephritis, pancreatitis, AAA
Low back pain with sciatica	Disc herniation, spinal stenosis, compression fracture, epidural abscess, intraspinal tumor/metastasis, vertebral osteomyelitis with compression fracture (late)
Low back pain without sciatica	Musculoligamentous, ankylosing spondylitis, spondylolisthesis, depression, vertebral osteomyelitis (early), epidural abscess (very early), retroperitoneal neoplasm

Investigations

Recommend:

- imaging: X-ray, CT, MRI, bone scan, US
- myelography, electromyography (EMG)
- immunoelectrophoresis

Management

For musculoskeletal neck pain:

- If there is instability or injury from a high risk trauma, immobilize the patient with a hard cervical collar until C-spines are cleared.
- Refer for surgery as needed.
- Administer muscle relaxants, nonnarcotic analgesia.
- Ensure early mobilization once instability excluded.
- Refer to physiotherapy.

For musculoskeletal back pain:

- Aim for early mobilization.
- Advise conservative bed rest (less than 4 days).
- Administer analgesics, muscle relaxants, NSAIDs.
- Refer to physiotherapy.
- Refer for surgical consult if:
  - o persistent disabling nerve root pain despite 4 to 6 weeks comprehensive conservative therapy
  - o neurologic deficits in the lower extremities
  - o disruption of bladder/bowel control

Case 131: Ankylosing spondylitis

A patient has been diagnosed with ankylosing spondylitis (AS). Please take a focused history, perform a focused physical exam, and recommend investigations.

Time: 10 minutes

History

Focus the history on issues specific to AS: family history, age, progression, uveitis, aortitis, and effects on breathing (chest expansion).

HISTORY OF PRESENT ILLNESS

Are your symptoms worse in the morning or later in the day? Do you have morning stiffness?

Do any of the following symptoms or factors apply to you? (See breakdown that follows.)

SYMPTOM/FACTOR	SYSTEM INVOLVED
Fever/chills, night sweats, weight loss, nocturnal pain, loss of appetite	Systemic
Inflammation of the eye (conjunctivitis, iritis, uveitis)	Ocular
Chest pain, palpitations	Cardiovascular (aortitis, aortic regurgitation)
Skin rashes, mouth ulcers	Cutaneous
Diarrhea, abdominal pain	GI
Painful urination (urethritis), diseases of the kidney (IgG nephropathy, amyloidosis)	GU
Joint pain (enthesitis, dactylitis, Achilles tendonitis)	Musculoskeletal
Swollen lymph nodes	Immune

PAST MEDICAL HISTORY

Do you have a history of any of the following?

- malignancy
- infections (TB)
- IV drug use
- recent genital or urinary procedures
- metabolic bone disease

Do any diseases run in your family? (Assess for HLA-B27 association.)

Physical exam

Focus the physical exam on issues specific to AS.

Assess:

- spine: occiput-to-wall distance, chest expansion, thoracic kyphosis, lumbar lordosis, ROM
- eyes, fingers, Achilles tendon

Perform a joint exam (see breakdown that follows).

JOINT	DETAILS
Hip	Inspect (patient supine):
	• alignment at rest, leg length (measure)
	Inspect (patient standing):
	• stance, swing, lumbar spine-lordosis, anterior-posterior of hip for muscle atrophy and bruising
	• gluteal fold (symmetry is important)
	• birth marks, hairy patch, surgical scars
	Palpate:
	• anterior-iliac crest, iliac tubercle, anterior superior iliac spine
	• posterior-superior iliac spine, greater trochanter, trochanteric bursa, ischial tuberosity, ischiogluteal bursa, sciatic nerve
	• front: inguinal ligament, including (mnemonic: **NAVEL**) **n**erve, **a**rtery, **v**ein, **e**mpty space, **l**ymph node; below ligament (ilial psoas bursa)
	Assess ROM:
	• abduction and flexion
	• exaggerated lordosis
	• internal and external rotation
	Do special tests:
	• Trendelenburg test: stand on affected leg, see if contralateral side drops or body leans over supported leg
	• straight-leg raise (sciatic nerve impingement)
	• Faber test (sacroiliac joint stress)
	• Ortolani/Barlow tests (pediatric)
Knee	Inspect:
	• gait, alignment and contour, hollows around patella
	• genus valgum or varum
	• bulk of quadriceps muscle (measure diameter)
	• effusion/joint swelling
	Palpate:
	• bone: medial/lateral femoral condyles, medial/lateral tibial plateaus, patella
	• muscle: quadriceps, patellar tendon, medial/lateral collateral ligaments
	• menisci and bursae: prepatellar, anserine bursa, semimembranosus bursa
	• joint effusion: milk sign, balloon sign, bulge sign, balloting sign
	Assess ROM:
	• stability, Lachman test, anterior/posterior drawer test
	• McMurray test for menisci

(Continued)

JOINT	DETAILS
Shoulder	Inspect:
	• contour, effusion, deformity, dislocation, muscle atrophy
	Palpate:
	• bones: clavicle, scapula, humerus, greater tubercle
	• joints: sternoclavicular (SC), scapulothoracic (ST), acromioclavicular (AC), glenohumeral (GH)
	• muscle: pectoralis major/minor, rotator cuff (supra/infraspinatus, teres minor, subscapularis), axioscapular group (trapezius, rhomboids, serratus anterior, levator scapula)
	• bursa: subacromial, axillary nerve distribution
	Assess ROM:
	• flexion, extension, external/internal rotation, abduction, adduction, ability to touch opposite shoulder, dropping sign
	• cervical: wing scapula (long thoracic nerve, muscle power)
	• passive versus active ROM
Elbow	Inspect:
	• alignment, swelling on either side of olecranon, olecranon bursa
	Palpate:
	• rheumatoid nodules, tennis/golfer elbow, ulnar nerve
	Assess ROM:
	• flexion, extension, supination, pronation
	• muscle: biceps, brachioradialis, triceps, supinator/pronator muscles

Investigations

Recommend:

- X-ray: bamboo spine, widening of sacroiliac (SI) joint, square lumbar spine
- ESR or CRP
- RF (negative in AS)

Case 132: Blocked Nose

A 60-year-old man says he has a blocked nose. Please obtain a focused history.

Time: 5 minutes

History

The history needs to establish whether the patient has prolonged blockage on one side (rule out tumor).

HISTORY OF PRESENT ILLNESS

How long has your nose been blocked?

Is it blocked on one side or both sides?

Is it blocked constantly or intermittently (e.g., variation with season)?

Does anything make your nose better or worse?

Do you have any of the following symptoms?

- nasal discharge, nosebleeds, headache, toothache
- weight loss, night sweats, loss of appetite, fever

PAST MEDICAL HISTORY

Have you had similar problems with your nose before? How was it treated? How did that go?

Have you had nasal surgery?

Do you have asthma or sensitivity to ASA?

What medications are you taking?

Do you use nasal drops? What kind? For how long? How frequently?

Does your family have a history of nasal tumors or other diseases (e.g., nasal polyps, allergic rhinitis, nasopharyngeal carcinoma)?

Do you sniff glue or illegal substances (cocaine)?

What is your ethnic background?

How old are you?

What is your occupation?

Case 133: Dysphagia

A 60-year-old woman is experiencing dysphagia. Please take a history, recommend investigations, and outline a management plan.

Time: 5 minutes

History

The history needs to establish whether the dysphagia is functional or structural, and esophageal or extraesophageal.

HISTORY OF PRESENT ILLNESS

What is your problem with swallowing like?

When did the problem start?

Did it develop gradually or suddenly? How has it changed since it began? Has it been intermittent or progressively worse?

Are you able to eat at all?

Can you move food to the back of mouth (i.e., initiate a swallow)?

Do you have trouble with solids, liquids, or both?

Is the problem different with hot versus cold food?

Does anything make the problem better or worse?

Do you have any of the following symptoms?

- pain when swallowing
- a feeling of food moving into your chest or abdomen
- sensation of a lump in the throat all the time
- regurgitation
- reflux symptoms (e.g., regurgitation into the mouth, heartburn)
- gurgles or bulges in the neck on drinking
- chest pain, back pain, weight loss, bone pain, headache, voice change
- respiratory symptoms
- halitosis

PAST MEDICAL HISTORY

Do you have a history of any of the following?

- gastroesophageal reflux disease
- peptic ulcer
- mood changes, depression, anxiety
- thyroid disease

- radiation treatments or exposure
- caustic ingestions (e.g., lye)
- connective tissue disease

What medications do you take?

Do any diseases run in your family (e.g., esophageal tumors, motility problems)?

Do you smoke, drink, or use recreational drugs?

Physical exam

Like the history, the physical exam needs to establish whether the dysphagia is functional or structural, and esophageal or extraesophageal.

Check the mouth, pharynx, neck, and respiratory system.

Differential diagnosis

See Table 40.

Table 40. DIFFERENTIAL DIAGNOSIS OF DYSPHAGIA

CATEGORY	POSSIBLE ETIOLOGY
Oral cavity	Viral ulcer, trauma, tumor, infection (Ludwig angina)
Oropharynx	Tonsillitis, retropharyngeal abscess
Hypopharynx	Trauma, thyroid tumor, foreign body, inflammation, neuromuscular
Esophageal	Trauma/perforation Obstruction: • intrinsic: hiatus hernia, tumor, corrosive esophagitis/stricture, esophageal web, foreign body, diverticulum • extrinsic: mediastinal abnormality, vascular compression
Motility	Achalasia, diffuse esophageal spasm, scleroderma, diabetic neuropathy

Some symptoms and factors also point to etiology (see breakdown that follows).

SYMPTOMS/FACTORS	ETIOLOGY
Trouble with liquids and solids	Achalasia
Trouble with solids, intermittent, elderly patient, with chest pain	Diffuse esophageal spasm
Anxiety, young patient	Lower esophageal ring
Trouble with solids, progressive, with weight loss, odynophagia	Carcinoma
Chronic heartburn	Peptic stricture

Investigations

Recommend, as appropriate:

- barium swallow (see Table 41 for interpretation)
- endoscopy plus biopsy
- manometry
- provocative testing: acid perfusion-Bernstein test; edrophonium testing
- 24 h esophageal pH and pressure monitoring
- bronchoscopy, mediastinoscopy

Table 41. BARIUM SWALLOW INTERPRETATION

ETIOLOGY	IDENTIFYING FEATURES
Peptic esophagitis	Prominent mucosal folds in distal esophagus
Peptic stricture	Smooth tapered narrowing
Diffuse spasm	Static contractile areas, poor propulsion, or lodging of solid food bolus
Carcinoma	Abrupt narrowing, sharp angulation of margins
Collagen disease (e.g., scleroderma)	Barium remains long after swallow
Achalasia	Dilated above sphincter, tortuous, poor emptying, bird's beak sign
Zenker diverticulum	Typical protruding pouch

Management

The treatment for achalasia/motility disorder includes (as appropriate):

- counseling the patient to eat slowly, drink small quantities at a time, and avoid cold foods
- a trial of sublingual nitrates or calcium channel blockers
- antireflux therapy
- antidepressants, relaxation techniques, behavioral methods
- esophageal dilatation, myotomy, botulinum toxin injections

The treatment for obstructive disorder includes, as appropriate:

- dilatation
- surgery
- radiation/chemotherapy
- nutrition changes

For infection, administer antibiotics, antifungals, or antivirals, as appropriate.

Abbreviations

3TC	lamivudine (2',3'-dideoxy-3'-thiacytidine)
AAA	abdominal aortic aneurysm
ABC	airway, breathing, circulation
ABG	arterial blood gas
ACE	angiotensin-converting enzyme
ADP	adenosine diphosphate
ALP	alkaline phosphatase
ALT	alanine transaminase
ANA	antinuclear antibody
ANCA	antineutrophil cytoplasmic antibodies
anti-HBc	hepatitis B core antibody
anti-HBe	hepatitis B envelope antibody
anti-HBs	hepatitis B surface antibody
ARB	angiotensin receptor blocker
ASA	acetylsalicylic acid
AST	aspartate transaminase
AZT	azidothymidine
BDZ	benzodiazepine
bid	twice a day
BP	blood pressure
BPH	benign prostatic hypertrophy
BUN	blood (serum) urea nitrogen
C&S	culture and sensitivity
C3	complement component 3
C4	complement component 4
Ca	calcium
CBC	complete blood count

CHF	congestive heart failure
CMV	cytomegalic virus
CNS	central nervous system
Cr	creatinine
CRP	C-reactive protein
CT	computed tomography
CXR	chest x-ray
D&C	dilation and curettage
D5W	dextrose 5% in water
DM	diabetes mellitus
DPB	diastolic blood pressure
DRE	digital rectal examination
ECG	electrocardiogram
EEG	electroencephalogram
EKG	electrocardiogram
ERCP	endoscopic retrograde cholangiopancreatography
ESR	erythrocyte sedimentation rate
FDP	fibrin degradation product
Fe	iron
FSH	follicle-stimulating hormone
GGT	gamma-glutamyl transpeptidase
GI	gastrointestinal
GU	genitourinary
HBcAg	hepatitis B core antigen
HBeAg	hepatitis B envelope antigen
HBIg	hepatitis B immunoglobulin
HBsAg	hepatitis B surface antigen
HBV	hepatitis B virus
hCG	human chorionic gonadotropin
HCV	hepatitis C virus
HEENT	head, ears, eyes, nose, throat
HIV	human immunodeficiency virus
HLA-B27	human leukocyte antigen B27
HTN	hypertension
HUS	hemolytic uremic syndrome
ICU	intensive care unit
IgA	α-immunoglobulin
IgG	gamma electrophoretic mobility
IM	intramuscular
INR	international normalized ratio
ITP	idiopathic thrombocytopenic purpura

IUD	intrauterine device
IV	intravenous
IVP	intravenous pyelogram
K	potassium
KCl	potassium chloride
KOH	potassium hydroxide
LFT	liver function test
LGV	lymphogranuloma venereum
LH	luteinizing hormone
LOC	level of consciousness
Mg	magnesium
MI	myocardial infarction
MRI	magnetic resonance imaging
NG	nasogastric
NS	normal saline
NSAID	nonsteroidal anti-inflammatory drug
po	by mouth (*per os*)
PTHrp	parathyroid hormone-related protein
PTT	partial thromboplastin time
q24h	every 24 hours (also, e.g., q6h)
ql	as necessary (*quantum libet*)
R/O	rule out
RBC	red blood cell
RF	rheumatoid factor
ROM	range of motion
RPR	rapid plasma reagin (test for syphilis)
SBP	systolic blood pressure
SLE	systemic lupus erythematosus
STD	sexually transmitted disease
TB	tuberculosis
TIBC	total iron building capacity
tid	3 times per day
TRUS	transrectal ultrasound
TSH	thyroid stimulating hormone
TTP	thrombotic thrombocytopenic purpura
TURP	transurethral resection of the prostate
URTI	upper respiratory tract infection
UTI	urinary tract infection
VDRL	venereal disease research laboratory (test for syphilis)

About the authors

Dr. Zu-hua Gao is a surgical pathologist with extensive clinical and teaching experience. He is currently Professor and Chair of the Department of Pathology at McGill University, and the Pathologist-in-Chief of McGill University Health Centre.

Dr. Christopher Naugler is a general pathologist and family physician with wide-ranging research, teaching, and clinical experience. He is an assistant professor in the Department of Pathology and Laboratory Medicine, and the Department of Family Medicine, at the University of Calgary, and with Calgary Laboratory Services.

List of cases

This list identifies the cases in the book by number only—so, without titles that identify etiology.

You can work through this list on your own, making notes on how you would handle each case and comparing them to the case notes in the book.

You can also use this list to practice clinical skills in groups. Groups of 3 or 4 work best, role-playing **candidate**, **examiner**, and **observer**(s). Candidates should read their cases from this list.

CASE 1

A 50-year-old woman presents with acidemia. Please recommend and explain appropriate investigations.

Time: 5 minutes

CASE 2

A 55-year-old man comes to your office angry because his insurance turned him down for abnormal liver-function tests. He wants you to "sort out this mistake." His tests to date show very high transaminases, slightly elevated alkaline phosphatase, and normal bilirubin. Please take a history, do a physical exam, provide a differential diagnosis, and recommend investigations.

Time: 10 minutes

CASE 3

A 40-year-old woman presents with jaundice. Please take a history.

Time: 5 minutes

CASE 4

A person with asthma comes to your office because she has had a cough for the past 2 weeks. Please take a focused history.

Time: 5 minutes

CASE 5

A 60-year-old man visits your office because he is worried about an aortic stenosis that was found by his family doctor, although he is currently asymptomatic. Please discuss condition management with the patient.

Time: 10 minutes

CASE 6

A 48-year-old woman has a critically high creatinine level. Please take a history, do a physical exam, and provide a differential diagnosis and key initial investigations.

Time: 10 minutes

CASE 7

A patient newly diagnosed with diabetes comes to you for advice on how to manage her condition.

Time: 5 minutes

CASE 8

A patient presents with diabetic ketoacidosis (DKA). Please obtain a focused history, do a physical exam, recommend investigations, and initiate appropriate management.

Time: 10 minutes

CASE 9

A 50-year-old university professor presents with a blood pressure reading of 160/98. He has undergone tests for HTN and had a physical examination, all of which had normal results. Please take a focused history and discuss with the patient how to manage his condition.

Time: 5 minutes

CASE 10

A young woman's routine physical examination for employment has shown abnormal hemoglobin and reticulocyte counts. Please take a history.

Time: 5 minutes

CASE 11

A 69-year-old man is experiencing fatigue, dizziness, and an unsteady gait. Lab results show the following: mean corpuscular volume (MCV) 120, hemoglobin (Hb) 90, white blood count 3.4. Please take a history, perform a focused physical exam, and determine what further investigations may be required.

Time: 10 minutes

CASE 12

A 55-year-old man presents with crushing retrosternal chest pain. His blood pressure is 110/80, and his heart rate is 180 and irregular. Please take a focused history, perform a physical exam, interpret the patient's ECG, and initiate appropriate management.

Time: 10 minutes

CASE 13

A patient presents with pneumonia and coughing. Perform a physical exam, interpret the patient's X-ray, and recommend appropriate management.

Time: 10 minutes

CASE 14

A patient presents with dyspnea and chest pain. Please perform a physical exam, provide a differential diagnosis, and recommend appropriate investigations.

Time: 10 minutes

CASE 15

A patient with a pulmonary embolism wants advice about anticoagulant use. Please take a history and discuss anticoagulant management with the patient.

Time: 5 minutes

CASE 16

A 60-year-old woman presents with paroxysmal atrial tachycardia while on digoxin. Her pulse is irregular on examination. She is concerned about taking digoxin, particularly because she plans to vacation in Florida soon. Please take a history and discuss the management of the patient's condition with digoxin.

Time: 5 minutes

CASE 17

A 60-year-old man is experiencing hemoptysis and shortness of breath. Please take a history and provide a management strategy.

Time: 5 minutes

CASE 18

A young woman presents with night sweats and lymphadenopathy, which comes and goes. Obtain a history, perform a physical exam, provide a differential diagnosis, and recommend investigations.

Time: 10 minutes

CASE 19

A 50-year-old woman presents with hilar adenopathy. Please give a differential diagnosis, and recommend and explain blood tests.

Time: 5 minutes

CASE 20

A 40-year-old woman presents with hypothyroidism. Please obtain a history, perform a physical exam, and provide a differential diagnosis.

Time: 10 minutes

CASE 21

A patient presents with elevated serum calcium. Please take a focused history, perform a physical exam, provide a differential diagnosis, and recommend relevant investigations and a plan for management.

Time: 10 minutes

CASE 22

A patient with a history of varicose veins has had claudication and calf pain for the past 6 months. Please perform a physical exam and interpret the patient's ECG. Give a differential diagnosis with risk factors, and recommend relevant investigations.

Time: 10 minutes

CASE 23

A 35-year-old man, who has been previously healthy other than obesity, is interested in losing weight. Please discuss management strategies with him.

Time: 5 minutes

CASE 24

A 35-year-old patient is experiencing fatigue. Please take a history, provide a differential diagnosis, recommend investigations, and outline a management plan.

Time: 10 minutes

CASE 25

A 21-year-old woman presents with a skin rash. Please obtain a focused history and perform a physical exam.

Time: 10 minutes

CASE 26

A patient is experiencing joint pain. Please take a history, do a physical exam, provide a differential diagnosis, and recommend relevant investigations.

Time: 10 minutes

CASE 27

A 40-year-old man is experiencing hair loss. Please take a history.

Time: 5 minutes

CASE 28

An 80-year-old man presents with recent weight loss. Please take a history, do a physical exam, and recommend investigations.

Time: 10 minutes

CASE 29

A 60-year-old woman visits your office because she has a sore throat. Please obtain a focused history.

Time: 5 minutes

CASE 30

A patient presents with bilateral ankle edema. Please take a history, do a physical exam, provide a differential diagnosis, recommend investigations, and outline an initial management strategy.

Time: 10 minutes

CASE 31

A patient with HIV needs treatment for recently diagnosed *Pneumocystis jiroveci*. Please perform a physical exam and outline a management strategy.

Time: 5 minutes

CASE 32

A 30-year-old woman has had repeated epistaxis and skin bruises. Please take a history, perform a physical exam, provide a differential diagnosis, and recommend investigations.

Time: 10 minutes

CASE 33

A patient presents with unilateral right hand weakness. Please take a history, provide a differential diagnosis, and recommend investigations.

Time: 5 minutes

CASE 34

A 30-year-old woman presents with amenorrhea. Please obtain a focused history and recommend investigations.

Time: 5 minutes

CASE 35

A 41-year-old woman has had heavy vaginal bleeding for the past 3 periods. Please take a history, provide a differential diagnosis, recommend investigations, and outline a management plan.

Time: 5 minutes

CASE 36

A 40-year-old woman presents with vaginal bleeding. Please obtain a history and provide a differential diagnosis.

Time: 5 minutes

CASE 37

A woman who is 7 weeks pregnant presents with vaginal bleeding and lower abdominal pain. Please obtain a focused history, provide a differential diagnosis with treatment options, and outline appropriate investigations.

Time: 5 minutes

CASE 38

A woman presents with bloody vaginal discharge. Please obtain a history, give a differential diagnosis, and recommend investigations.

Time: 5 minutes

CASE 39

A 37-year-old woman is 9 weeks pregnant and concerned about trisomy 21. Please take a history and discuss a management plan with her.

Time: 5 minutes

CASE 40

A 24-year-old woman is pregnant, but she doesn't want to give birth to a child at this time in her life. Please take a history and discuss a management strategy with the patient.

Time: 10 minutes

CASE 41

A woman who is 36 to 40 weeks pregnant presents with proteinuria and a blood pressure reading of 130/85 (from 110/65). Please take a history, provide a differential diagnosis, and outline a management plan.

Time: 10 minutes

CASE 42

A 20-year-old pregnant woman presents with lower left quadrant (LLQ) pain. Please take a focused history, perform a physical exam, give a differential diagnosis, and propose investigations.

Time: 5 minutes

CASE 43

A 25-year-old woman who is pregnant has concerns about breast-feeding. Please take a history and discuss a management plan with her.

Time: 5 minutes

CASE 44

A 20-year-old woman is pregnant with her second child. She had a C-section with her first child due to fetal distress. She is concerned about having another C-section.

Time: 5 minutes

CASE 45

A 20-year-old woman requests birth control pills. Please take a history and counsel her.

Time: 5 minutes

CASE 46

A 37-year-old woman, who has been married for 7 years, presents with infertility. Please obtain a focused history.

Time: 5 minutes

CASE 47

A 75-year-old woman presents with incontinence. Please take a history and provide a differential diagnosis.

Time: 5 minutes

CASE 48

A 2-year-old girl has developed a cough after being on antibiotics. Please obtain a history and provide a differential diagnosis.

Time: 5 minutes

CASE 49

A 1-year-old boy has had diarrhea for 6 months. Please obtain a history, provide a differential diagnosis, and recommend investigations.

Time: 5 minutes

CASE 50

A father comes to see you because he believes his child is hyperactive. Please obtain a history and discuss a management plan with the father.

Time: 5 minutes

CASE 51

The parents of a 3-year-old girl are worried about her development. Her speech is far behind others in her age group. She only says "mom" and "dad." Compared to her older brother, she has been slower to achieve development milestones. Please obtain a history and give a differential diagnosis.

Time: 5 minutes

CASE 52

A 6-year-old girl presents with dysphrasia. Please take a history and assess her status.

Time: 10 minutes

CASE 53

An infant boy presents with failure to thrive. Please take a history and discuss a management strategy with the mother.

Time: 5 minutes

CASE 54

A mother phones your office in distress because her 18-month-old son has swallowed some antihypertensive medication. Please give her advice over the phone and outline a management plan for the emergency room.

Time: 5 minutes

CASE 55

A 6-week-old infant presents with a 3-day history of vomiting. Please take a history and recommend investigations.

Time: 5 minutes

CASE 56

A mother comes to your office with her adolescent son, who is using drugs. She is seeking your advice on what to do. Please take a history and outline a management plan.

Time: 10 minutes

CASE 57

A teenager with a history of epilepsy has been experiencing increased seizures. Please take a history and outline a management strategy.

Time: 5 minutes

CASE 58

The parents of a 12-month-old boy have noted that their son seems pale. Please take a focused history and provide a differential diagnosis

Time: 5 minutes

CASE 59

A child has diarrhea with bloody stools. Please obtain a history.

Time: 10 minutes

CASE 60

A mother comes to your office because her 18-month-old daughter has had a seizure accompanied by a high fever. Please take a history and discuss a management plan with the mother.

Time: 5 minutes

CASE 61

A parent brings an injured child to you. You suspect physical abuse. Please obtain a history, do a physical exam, and outline a management plan.

Time: 10 minutes

CASE 62

An infant girl presents with jaundice 48 hours after birth. Please obtain a history from the mother and provide a differential diagnosis.

Time: 5 minutes

CASE 63

A newborn baby has delayed passage of meconium. Please provide a differential diagnosis and outline a management plan, including investigations.

Time: 5 minutes

CASE 64

A 6-year-old girl has pain on micturition. You suspect sexual abuse. Please obtain a history from the mother and outline a strategy for management.

Time: 5 minutes

CASE 65

A 45-year-old woman has delivered a low-birth-weight baby. Please obtain a focused history, and provide a differential diagnosis that lists complications.

Time: 5 minutes

CASE 66

A 15-year-old girl wants advice about her acne. Please take a history and discuss a management plan with her.

Time: 5 minutes

CASE 67

A patient has been sexually assaulted. Please take a history.

Time: 5 minutes

CASE 68

A 30-year-old woman wants to learn how to do a breast self-exam. Please counsel her.

Time: 5 minutes

CASE 69

A 30-year-old woman is seeking advice because her mother and 2 sisters have all had breast cancer. Please take a history, recommend appropriate investigations, and discuss a management plan with her.

Time: 5 minutes

CASE 70

A 30-year-old man is experiencing erectile dysfunction. Please take a history, provide a differential diagnosis, and recommend investigations.

Time: 5 minutes

CASE 71

A 28-year-old man presents with penile discharge. Please obtain a history, perform a physical exam, provide a differential diagnosis, and recommend investigations.

Time: 10 minutes

CASE 72

A new immigrant mother wants information about immunizing her baby. Please take a history and discuss a management plan with her.

Time: 5 minutes

CASE 73

An elderly man has made an appointment because he has experienced 2 falls. The man's son has accompanied him to the appointment, and is concerned about injury to his father from falling and about his father's mobility. Please take a history, provide a differential diagnosis, and recommend investigations.

Time: 5 minutes

CASE 74

A nurse has had a needle-stick injury from a source patient who was HBsAg positive and HIV negative. Please take a history and discuss a management plan with the patient.

Time: 5 minutes

CASE 75

A woman has been physically assaulted by her partner. Please take a history and outline a management plan.

Time: 10 minutes

CASE 76

A woman who has recently emigrated has had a chest X-ray as part of a screening process for her work. The X-ray is abnormal. Please take a history and provide a differential diagnosis.

Time: 5 minutes

CASE 77

A 20-year-old man is experiencing severe mood swings. His concerned sister has accompanied him to his appointment. Please take a history and outline a management plan.

Time: 10 minutes

CASE 78

The wife of a 25-year-old man has brought her husband to you because he is experiencing anxiety. Please obtain a history.

Time: 5 minutes

CASE 79

A 50-year-old woman, who had a hysterectomy 3 days ago, says she is hearing music and feels insects crawling on her. Please obtain a history and provide a mental disorder assessment.

Time: 10 minutes

CASE 80

An elderly woman is experiencing multiple aches and pains. She has been seen by many physicians and has been extensively investigated with no diagnosis. She has seen your partner in your clinic and was not satisfied with their assessment, and so has come to you. Please take a history and discuss a management plan with the patient.

Time: 10 minutes

CASE 81

A mother brings her 16-year-old daughter to see you because she is concerned about her daughter's recent weight loss. You suspect anorexia nervosa. Please take a history, do a metal status exam (MSE), and discuss a management plan with the patient and her mother.

Time: 10 minutes

CASE 82

A young woman comes to you because she feels down. Please take a history, provide a differential diagnosis, and outline a management plan.

Time: 5 minutes

CASE 83

A 20-year-old man has attempted suicide by ingesting ASA. He is in hospital and medically cleared. Please do a psychiatric assessment.

Time: 5 minutes

CASE 84

A patient is suspected of having taken an overdose of sleeping pills. Please initiate appropriate management.

Time: 5 minutes

CASE 85

An 18-year-old patient presents with a seizure disorder and an increased number of seizures. Please take a history, do a physical exam, recommend investigations, and discuss a management plan with the patient.

Time: 10 minutes

CASE 86

A 35-year-old man with a history of alcoholism has just had a convulsion. Please perform a physical exam.

Time: 10 minutes

CASE 87

A 60-year-old man presents with difficulty walking. Please do a focused physical exam and provide a differential diagnosis.

Time: 5 minutes

CASE 88

A 60-year-old man presents with a tremor in his hands. Please take a focused history and do a focused physical exam to assess him for Parkinson disease.

Time: 5 minutes

CASE 89

A teenage patient has had a recent URTI. For the last 2 days, the patient has been experiencing fever, vomiting, headache, and drowsiness. Please do a physical exam, provide a differential diagnosis, and recommend investigations.

Time: 10 minutes

CASE 90

A comatose patient is brought to the emergency room. Please initiate appropriate management.

Time: 5 minutes

CASE 91

An elderly patient presents with decreased memory and increased confusion. Please take a history, perform a neurological exam, and outline a management plan.

Time: 10 minutes

CASE 92

A 58-year-old man presents with dysphasia. Please take a history and assess his status.

Time: 10 minutes

CASE 93

A 50-year-old woman had a hysterectomy 4 days ago. She is now experiencing auditory and visual hallucinations. She was recently given Tylenol 3 and Ativan 1 mg. Please take a focused history and conduct an appropriate examination.

Time: 5 minutes

CASE 94

A patient has a neck injury. Please perform a neurological assessment.

Time: 5 minutes

CASE 95

A 60-year-old woman comes to the emergency room with new-onset left-sided hemiparesis and right-sided facial droop. Please take a history, perform a physical exam, provide a differential diagnosis, recommend investigations, and outline a management plan.

Time: 10 minutes

CASE 96

A 65-year-old man comes to your office with his wife. She says her husband is becoming hard of hearing. Please take a history, give a differential diagnosis, and recommend investigations.

Time: 5 minutes

CASE 97

A 40-year-old woman says she is having difficulty sleeping. Please take a history, do a physical exam, recommend investigations, and discuss a management plan with the patient.

Time: 5 minutes

CASE 98

A 50-year-old man who is a heavy smoker has come to you for advice on how to quit smoking. Please discuss a management plan with the patient.

Time: 10 minutes

CASE 99

An alcoholic has been charged with drunk driving and wants help to stop drinking. Please take a history and discuss a management plan with the patient.

Time: 10 minutes

CASE 100

A 55-year-old woman says she feels a lump in her throat when she swallows. Please take a focused history.

Time: 5 minutes

CASE 101

A 70-year-old man is experiencing visual disturbances. Please take a focused history.

Time: 5 minutes

CASE 102

A 55-year-old man has a hoarse voice. Please take a history, provide a differential diagnosis, and recommend investigations.

Time: 5 minutes

CASE 103

A 35-year-old man presents with dizziness. Please take a focused history, do a physical exam, provide a differential diagnosis, and recommend investigations.

Time: 10 minutes

CASE 104

A patient presents with a history of headache. Please obtain a history, perform a physical exam, provide a differential diagnosis, recommend investigations, and outline a management plan.

Time: 10 minutes

CASE 105

A 20-year-old man from out of town wants Fiorinal for headaches. Please take a history and discuss a management plan with the patient.

Time: 5 minutes

CASE 106

A 60-year-old woman presents with nipple discharge. Her mammogram shows microcalcification. Please take a history and discuss a management plan with the patient.

Time: 5 minutes

CASE 107

A patient presents with wrist pain and finger numbness. Please take a history, do a focused physical exam, provide a differential diagnosis, recommend investigations, and outline a management strategy.

Time: 10 minutes

CASE 108

A patient presents with acute abdominal pain. Please do a physical exam, provide a differential diagnosis, and recommend investigations.

Time: 10 minutes

CASE 109

A 40-year-old man comes to the emergency room with agonizing abdominal pain. Please carry out the necessary examination and provide a differential diagnosis. Initiate appropriate management.

Time: 5 minutes

CASE 110

A middle-aged woman presents with a thyroid mass. Please obtain a history, do a focused physical exam, and recommend investigations.

Time: 5 minutes

CASE 111

A 20-year-old man presents with an ankle injury. Please assess the injury, recommend investigations, and initiate appropriate management.

Time: 5 minutes

CASE 112

A 20-year-old man has been stabbed in the epigastrium. His blood pressure reading is 90/40. Please initiate appropriate management.

Time: 5 minutes

CASE 113

A 30-year-old man has fallen from a height of 10 meters. He presents with tenderness in the left upper quadrant (LUQ) and a wound on the left leg. He has a neck collar on but wants it removed. He wants analgesics. Please initiate appropriate management.

Time: 10 minutes

CASE 114

A patient has suffered a head trauma in a motor vehicle collision. Please initiate appropriate management.

Time: 10 minutes

CASE 115

A 20-year-old man has lacerated his right forearm on a broken beer bottle. Please obtain a history, do a physical exam, and initiate appropriate management.

Time: 10 minutes

CASE 116

A burn victim comes to the emergency room. Please initiate appropriate management.

Time: 10 minutes

CASE 117

An 18-year-old man is experiencing testicular pain. Please take a focused history, do a focused physical exam, provide a differential diagnosis, and recommend investigations.

Time: 5 minutes

CASE 118

A 60-year-old man says he has a bulge in the groin. Please take a history, do a physical exam, recommend investigations, and outline a management plan.

Time: 5 minutes

CASE 119

A 60-year-old woman presents with a breast lump. Please obtain a history, recommend investigations, and provide appropriate management.

Time: 5 minutes

CASE 120

A 60-year-old man has been unable to urinate for 12 hours. Please obtain a history, provide a differential diagnosis, and recommend investigations.

Time: 5 minutes

CASE 121

A patient presents with lower GI bleeding. Please take a history, give a differential diagnosis, and initiate appropriate management.

Time: 5 minutes

CASE 122

An adult patient presents with vomiting of several days duration. Please take a focused history.

Time: 5 minutes

CASE 123

A 50-year-old woman says she is experiencing chronic constipation. Please take a focused history and suggest investigations.

Time: 5 minutes

CASE 124

A 70-year-old woman has had diarrhea since discharge from hospital 10 days ago. Please take a focused history and suggest investigations.

Time: 5 minutes

CASE 125

A patient presents with hematemesis. Please initiate appropriate management.

Time: 5 minutes

CASE 126

A routine chest X-ray reveals a nodule in a 50-year-old female patient. Please perform a focused physical exam, provide a differential diagnosis, and recommend investigations.

Time: 5 minutes

CASE 127

A 50-year-old smoker and current textile worker has a likely diagnosis of lung cancer. Please discuss a management plan with the patient.

Time: 5 minutes

CASE 128

An 80-year-old woman is brought to the emergency room by her granddaughter. She is unconscious with a heart rate of 40 and a blood pressure reading of 80/40. Please initiate appropriate management and provide a differential diagnosis.

Time: 10 minutes

CASE 129

A routine urinalysis on a 50-year-old man reveals an RBC count of 50. Please take a history, perform a physical exam, provide a differential diagnosis, and recommend investigations.

Time: 10 minutes

CASE 130

A patient is experiencing neck pain. Please take a history, perform a physical exam, provide a differential diagnosis, and outline a management plan.

Time: 10 minutes

CASE 131

A patient has been diagnosed with ankylosing spondylitis (AS). Please take a focused history, perform a focused physical exam, and recommend investigations.

Time: 10 minutes

CASE 132

A 60-year-old man says he has a blocked nose. Please obtain a focused history.

Time: 5 minutes

CASE 133

A 60-year-old woman is experiencing dysphagia. Please take a history, recommend investigations, and outline a management plan.

Time: 5 minutes

Index of cases
by page number